MIX
Papier aus verantwortungsvollen Quellen
Paper from responsible sources
FSC® C105338

Azza El Amir

Parasitic Antigens for Vaccine Development

Anchor Academic
Publishing

El Amir, Azza: Parasitic Antigens for Vaccine Development, Hamburg, Anchor Academic Publishing 2016

Buch-ISBN: 978-3-96067-054-4
PDF-eBook-ISBN: 978-3-96067-554-9
Druck/Herstellung: Anchor Academic Publishing, Hamburg, 2016

Bibliografische Information der Deutschen Nationalbibliothek:
Die Deutsche Nationalbibliothek verzeichnet diese Publikation in der Deutschen Nationalbibliografie; detaillierte bibliografische Daten sind im Internet über http://dnb.d-nb.de abrufbar.

Bibliographical Information of the German National Library:
The German National Library lists this publication in the German National Bibliography. Detailed bibliographic data can be found at: http://dnb.d-nb.de

All rights reserved. This publication may not be reproduced, stored in a retrieval system or transmitted, in any form or by any means, electronic, mechanical, photocopying, recording or otherwise, without the prior permission of the publishers.

Das Werk einschließlich aller seiner Teile ist urheberrechtlich geschützt. Jede Verwertung außerhalb der Grenzen des Urheberrechtsgesetzes ist ohne Zustimmung des Verlages unzulässig und strafbar. Dies gilt insbesondere für Vervielfältigungen, Übersetzungen, Mikroverfilmungen und die Einspeicherung und Bearbeitung in elektronischen Systemen.

Die Wiedergabe von Gebrauchsnamen, Handelsnamen, Warenbezeichnungen usw. in diesem Werk berechtigt auch ohne besondere Kennzeichnung nicht zu der Annahme, dass solche Namen im Sinne der Warenzeichen- und Markenschutz-Gesetzgebung als frei zu betrachten wären und daher von jedermann benutzt werden dürften.

Die Informationen in diesem Werk wurden mit Sorgfalt erarbeitet. Dennoch können Fehler nicht vollständig ausgeschlossen werden und die Diplomica Verlag GmbH, die Autoren oder Übersetzer übernehmen keine juristische Verantwortung oder irgendeine Haftung für evtl. verbliebene fehlerhafte Angaben und deren Folgen.

Alle Rechte vorbehalten

© Anchor Academic Publishing, Imprint der Diplomica Verlag GmbH
Hermannstal 119k, 22119 Hamburg
http://www.diplomica-verlag.de, Hamburg 2016
Printed in Germany

Abstract

Despite effective chemotherapy, fascioliasis remains a major public health problem in developing world, with at least 17 million active infections resulting in significant morbidity, late infection detection and rapid reinfection after treatment, mandates alternative control strategies. Proteases, a myofibrillar protein, found only in invertebrates. In the present study, adult fresh *Fasciola gigantica* (*F. gigantica*) worms were homogenized; Antigen was purified and used to raise rabbit polyclonal antibodies (pAb). The purified pAb was then used in sandwich ELISA to detect *Fasciola* antigens in sera samples from a total 135 cattle. Sandwich ELISA showed 97.33% sensitivity and 95% specificity, in comparison to parasitological investigation that showed only 66.66% sensitivity and 100% specificity, respectively. Also, we demonstrated that mixed Th1/Th2 immune response to Antigen is associated with resistance to fascioliasis infection. We developed an experimental model of *F. gigantica* with rabbits, and use it to evaluate vaccination strategy with antigen. Twelve-week-old rabbits successfully infected by dermal penetration of 25 *F. gigantica* metacercariae, showing 58.40% worm recovery and 61.40% bile egg reduction. Examination of immunoglobulin M (IgM) and total IgG in serum and the cytokine profile, represented a predominance of IgG2 isotype indicating Th1 response which characterized by cellular immunity, and reveals production of interleukin-10 (IL-10) that initiate Th2 response. In conclusion, Antigen is presented as a promising antigen in early immunodiagnosis and a vaccine candidate for protection against fascioliasis infection.

Keywords: *F. gigantica*, Antigen, pAb, immunodiagnosis, vaccine, cytokines, Igs.

CONTENTS

	Page
INTRODUCTION	5
REVIEW OF LITERATURE	7
MATERIALS AND METHODS	29
RESULTS	36
DISCUSSION	41
REFERENCES	50

Introduction

Fascioliasis and other plant-borne trematodes zoonoses are well known helminths parasites of herbivorous animals which is caused by two trematodes *F. hepatica* and *F. gigantica*. This disease is found in many areas as Europe, the Americans, Africa and Asia, which results in major economic losses in agriculture communities **(Mas-Coma et al., 2005)**.

Fascioliasis reduces the production of meat, milk and wool, in addition to losses due to mortalities, liver condemnation and expenditures for antihelminthic using **(Awad et al., 2009)**. Human infection with fascioliasis is reported according to world health organization **(WHO, 2007)**. In Egypt fascioliasis, existed since Pharaonic ages **(Soliman, 2008)**, can infect also donkeys and camels as well as herbivorous animals, which will finally infect human leading to serious hepatic pathological sequences. About 830.000 people are infected in Egypt **(WHO, 1995)**. The clinical manifestations of fascioliasis in humans include fever, abdominal pain, persistent diarrhea, vomiting and Eosinophilia. Fascioliasis can be differentially diagnosed from some other diseases as acute hepatitis, schistosomiasis, visceral toxocariasis, biliary tract diseases and hepatic amoebiasis **(Keyyu et al., 2006; Ganga et al., 2007)**. Treatment of the disease for human is WHO major concern, using Tric labendazole (TCBZ) which is effective at single dose in Egypt **(Soliman, 2008)**. Despite that chemotherapy with TCBZ is effective in treatment, it does not prevent reinfection. Therefore, animals in endemic countries must be continuously treated with the drug. This approach is prohibitively expensive for developing countries and furthermore, promotes the threat of drug resistance **(Barduagni et al., 2008)**.

Thus, prevention and control of the disease is important to provide a proper treatment before liver damage occurs; this will be achieved by early diagnosis of the disease and development of a proper vaccine for prophylaxis from infection **(Intapan et al., 2003)**.

The parasitological diagnosis of fascioliasis is based on identification of eggs in stool, duodenal contents or bile, also by recovery of the adult worm during surgical exploration (after treatment) or at autopsy. However, the eggs may be absent or present in very small number at irregular intervals, hence difficult to be found. Besides, the eggs may be transiently present in stool after ingestion of raw or uncooked liver from infected animals. The symptoms of fascioliasis may be present for several weeks (wk) before eggs are recovered in stool. Thus, serologic tests are alternative methods of confirming fascioliasis. However, cross-reactions with other helminthic antigens may confuse the interpretation of the results **(Haseeb et al., 2002)**. But detection of circulating antigens is more specific using antibodies due to no cross reactivity with other parasites **(Bossaert et al., 2000)**.

Several antigens are needed for efficient diagnostic methods and/or vaccine preparation. Proteases a fibrillar membrane protein widely distributed among invertebrates but absent in vertebrates, was defined as a potential candidate antigen to develop vaccines against some helminthiases, i.e. schistosomiasis and filariasis. Several vaccination trials are under way, or have been conducted, using either the native or recombinant protein. Different levels of response and protection have been achieved in animals **(Cancela *et al.*, 2004)**.

This work aims to evaluate an early immunodiagnosis protocol for fascioliasis using sandwich ELISA to Antigen. On the other hand, study the humoral and cellular immune response for developing a vaccine using *F. gigantica* Antigen which is isolated from adult worm homogenate during parasite invasion to give protection against this disease.

Review of Literature

Fascioliasis may lead to economic losses of weight gain, fertility and milk production, in case of infection with *F. hepatica*, ovine fascioliasis can result in significant blood loss, representing a loss of metabolizable energy. This together with impaired appetite can have an adverse effect on weight gain, the greatest reduction in weight gain occurred in first 16 week (wk) of infection and there is still a significant decrease in weight gain during chronic stage of the disease **(Torgerson and Claxton, 1999)**.

Goat fascioliasis is considered less frequent and less important than sheep and cattle infection; however, fascioliasis occurs as a major constraint for goat production in many areas of the world. It is known that the course of fascioliasis in the host varies according to the ruminant species; for example, fascioliasis is often chronic and subclinical in cattle, but acute and accompanied by high mortality in sheep **(Soulsby, 1982)**. Furthermore, the response against the parasite differs in different host species. Humans are usually infected by ingestion of leafy plants that contain infective metacercariae **(Mas-Coma *et al.*, 1999)**.

Epidemiology of the infection with *F. gigantica* is similar to that with *F. hepatica*, because the two parasites infect the liver of herbivorous animals and have similar forms of life cycle. Social and agricultural differences between tropical and temperate regions where *F. gigantica* and *F. hepatica* are endemic are considered as important differences that separate between the epidemiology of the two parasites **(Spithill *et al.*, 1997)**.

In Egypt, **Haridy *et al.* (1999)** reported that, during the years 1994 to 1997 the overall slaughtered animals in Egyptian abattoirs was 2,003,200 sheep and goats, 2,624,239 cattle and 3,536,744 buffaloes. The overall rates of fascioliasis were 2.02 % for sheep and goats, 3.54 % for cattle and 1.58 % for buffaloes. Macroscopic examination of sheep liver showed up to 100 flukes per liver inside largely dilated thick walled bile ducts. Cattle liver showed up to 275 flukes per liver inside thickened dilated and calcareous bile ducts with offensive yellowish brown bile. Buffalo's liver showed up to 330 flukes per liver. Microscopic examination showed mainly thickened wall, hyperplasia and marked fibrosis.

Eggs of *Fasciola* passed from bile duct into duodenum and later into feces. Eggs are composed of large number of yolk granules surrounding the fertilized ovum (140 μm long). When, these eggs are passed out into feces. They undergo embryonation, operculate and consist of two types of cells, somatic cell, which develops into the succeeding stage (miracidia), and germ or propagative cell responsible for the formation of the following stage outside the host, where they are exposed to several physio-chemical factors as temperature, humidity, and oxygen tension **(Andrews, 1999)**.

Miracidium escapes the egg within 1-2 wk in water, where it infects the snail as an intermediate host, *Lymnaea spp*. The penetration process involves a mechanical boring to the snail, which is facilitated by secretion of proteolytic enzymes, the time required for the development of miracidia in the eggs varies with temperature, 10-11 days at 37-38°C, 21-24 days at 25°C and 33 days at 17-22°C **(Garcia, 2001)**. Eggs do not survive at temperatures higher than 43-44°C **(Spithill *et al.*, 1999a)**. Eggs of *F. gigantica* do not all develop at the same rate so that, from the same batch, miracidia may hatch over a period up to 14 wk, thus enhancing their opportunity to infect a snail **(Guralp *et al.*, 1964)**. Once miracidia released from the egg, they survive in water for 18-26 hour (hr) **(Asanji, 1988)**. When the miracidium reaches its proper host, it adheres to its body by the apical papilla and penetrates its tissues, finding its way to the blood spaces in the roof of the pulmonary cavity **(Soliman, 1996)**.

Within the intermediate host, it develops into sporocyst **(Agarwal, 2003)**. Each sporocyst gives rise to 5-8 rediae that developed later into cercariae. The later leave the snail in 4-7 wk from the time of infection **(Soulsby, 1973)**, The cercariae has an oval body and a long unforked tail (leptocercous); the body possesses a small anterior sucker surrounding the mouth, a large ventral sucker, a pharynx, a short esophagus and a two branched intestine in addition to rudiments of the genital organs **(Soliman, 1996)**. Cercariae are shed in up to 15 waves (usually three or fewer), 1-8 days apart over a period of about 7-50 days, in each wave, 50-70 cercariae are released **(Da-Costa *et al.*, 1994)**. Shedding commences as early as 20 days post infection (PI) of snails **(Sharma *et al.*, 1989)**. About 80% of cercariae are shed at night **(Da-Costa *et al.*, 1994)**. Cercariae swim for some days and eventually attach to aquatic grass blades. After losing the tail, they become encysted within a chitinous shell secreted by the cystogenous glands, thus changing into metacercariae (the infective stage). They can withstand adverse conditions for a wk **(Agarwal, 2003)**. About two-thirds attach to objects within 6.4 cm of the surface of the water **(Ueno and Yoshihara, 1974)**, and the remainders do not attach but become floating cysts **(Spithill *et al.*, 1999a)**.

The proportion of floating cysts is higher for *F. gigantica* than for *F. hepatica* **(Dreyfuss and Rondelaud, 1997)**. Newly encysted metacercariae requires at least 24 hr to become infective **(Boray, 1969)**, and when swallowed by the definitive host, the metacercariae excysts in the small intestine **(Dixon, 1966)**, where the cyst wall dissolves by the effect of the intestinal enzymes. The newly encysted juveniles (NEJs) penetrate intestinal mucosa, and then they develop into young flukes, bore their way through the wall of the host's intestine and migrate to the peritoneal cavity. After 3-5 days of wandering, they enter the liver causing serious damage to the hepatic tissue, or they may enter the bile ducts directly from the intestine or through the blood circulation. They become sexually mature within 2-3 months **(Soliman, 1996)**.

Human infection with fascioliasis can result from ingestion of encysted metacercariae attached to aquatic vegetation and plants **(Ragab and Farag, 1978)**. Eating raw or incompletely cooked crab or Cray fish, or by accidental transfer of cyst to mouth after handling raw vegetables, crabs or cray fish during preparation of food **(Yokogawa, 1982)**. Drinking of contaminated water with encysted metacercariae might be another way of infection, on the other hand, consuming raw liver dishes prepared from fresh livers infected with immature *F. gigantica* that lead to acute and chronic disease characterized by clinical symptoms as anorexia, fever and weight loss **(Taira et al., 1997)**.

The metacercarial larvae of *Fasciola* escape from cysts in duodenum and cause no significant damage as they migrate through duodenum wall into peritoneal cavity. When young migrating flukes reached the liver parenchyma, they cause traumatic and necrotic lesions due to heavily infiltration with eosinophils (Eo) **(Arora, 2005)**. The major pathological changes are seen during migration of these young flukes through liver parenchyma before they enter biliary tract. They digest the hepatic tissue and cause intensive hemorrhagic lesions, inflammatory reactions, and destruction of liver tissue and inflammation of bile ducts **(Marsden and Warren, 1984)**. While, less pathogenic effect to liver can be found when small numbers of flukes reach the bile duct, leading to inflammation and fibrosis of the bile duct **(Smithers and Doenhoff, 1982)**. When larvae reach the bile duct, it develops into adult and causes gastrointestinal symptoms. Some patients develop chronic cholecystitis, cholangitis and cholilithiasis, which may be accompanied by biliary colic, epigastric pain, jaundice, nausea, pruritis and upper right quadrant pain. In heavy infections, young worms may wonder back into liver parenchyma producing abscesses. Larvae migrating through peritoneal cavity may become lodged in ectopic foci, where abscesses or fibrotic lesions may develop. These sites include blood vessels, lungs, subcutaneous tissue, ventricles of brain **(Arora, 2005)**.

Consequences of liver damage resulting from the migrating flukes compromises liver function which is reflected in changes of plasma protein concentration (albumin and globulin). Changes of levels of hepatic enzymes released into the blood as a result of liver tissue damage are used as monitor to progress of infection and sensitive diagnostic aid in field infection **(Gajewska et al., 2005)**. A decrease in hemoglobin, packed cell volume, total erythrocyte counts and appearance of reticulocytes in blood of *F. gigantica* infected buffaloes to hypothyroidism **(Ganga et al., 2007)**. Most patients with fascioliasis develop cell-mediated immune response and specific antibodies against *Fasciola* worms. This specific humoral immune response could be followed by formation of localized or circulating immune complex

(CIC), which could be involved in the immunological mechanism of host-fluke relationship **(Shaker et al., 1994)**. Human fascioliasis is considered as a serious hepatic pathological threat to livers of Egyptian population, where it is diagnosed from some diseases as acute hepatitis, initial symptoms most frequently include severe headache, chills and fever. Enlarged tender or cirrhotic liver accompanied by diarrhea and anemia indicates advanced infection **(Keyyu et al., 2006)**.

1. Pathology

A. In human

The clinical picture of fascioliasis is usually divided into three major forms:

- **Acute Fascioliasis:** It corresponds to the migratory phase of the NEJs in the liver and occurs within 2-3 months after acquiring the infection. Fever, abdominal pain, headache, pruritis, urticaria, weight loss, and Eosinophilia. Transaminase levels are in normal range or are only minimally elevated, and bilirubin levels are typically in normal range **(Patil et al., 2009)**.

- **Chronic Fascioliasis:** It corresponds to the presence of mature adult parasites in bile ducts inside the liver and symptoms begin about 1 month after the exposure to metacercariae, are fever, general malaise, fatigue, hepatomegaly, anorexia, weight loss, urticaria with dermatographism and peripheral blood Eosinophilia. The symptoms may be absent in cases of light infection. The biliary phase may be asymptomatic or there may be symptoms related to cholangitis and obstruction of the biliary tract due to the enlarging fluke(s). The biliary phase may last for months or years **(Kanoksil et al., 2006)**.

- **Ectopic Fascioliasis:** It is found in organs and subcutaneous tissues in the abdominal region. They were also found in lungs, heart, eyes, brain, and lymph nodes. This is due to secondary infection in the liver by clostridium species occurring in necrotic hemorrhagic lesions produced by young parasites migrating within the liver **(Cho et al., 1994)**. Also, rarely, a condition known as "black disease" occurs as a complication of fascioliasis **(Boray, 1999)**.

B. In animals

The clinical picture of fascioliasis is usually divided into three major stages:

- **Pre-hepatic stage**: It is associated with the least pathology but sheep may experience ascites, pneumonia and fibrous pleuritis. Other signs include edema "bottle jaw" **(Behm and Sangster, 1999)**.

- **Hepatic or parenchymal stage:** It is associated with immature flukes burrowing through the liver. Clinical signs are preferable to hepatitis and include signs referable to derangement of amino acid metabolism, carbohydrate and lipid balance, urea synthesis, detoxification metabolism, ketogenesis and albumin and glutathione synthesis. Clinical signs include inappetance, ill-thrift, abdominal pain, jaundice, anemia, weakness, respiratory distress and collapse. Hepatic fibrosis and calcification may occur as a result of chronic infection, particularly in less permissible hosts like cattle and humans **(Behm and Sangster, 1999)**.

- Post-hepatic stage: It is associated with the establishment of adult flukes in the bile ducts where they become patent. This occurs approximately 7 to 8 wk PI. Little inflammatory response occurs once flukes are established in the bile duct, however bile duct hypertrophy and calcification is not uncommon in cattle or humans. The presence of a large number of flukes can mechanically obstruct bile ducts **(Smyth, 1994; Andrews, 1999; Behm and Sangster, 1999)**.

Economical effect of fascioliasis in sheep is due to sudden deaths of animals as well as reduction of weight gain and wool production. In goats and cattle, the clinical manifestation is similar to sheep. However, acquired resistance to *F. hepatica* infection is well-known in adult cattle **(Behm and Sangster, 1999; Boray, 1999)**.

2. Immune Response Against Fasciola

Whether, the immune responses which develop in humans in response to liver and lung fluke infections confer protective immunity against the currently held parasites or NEJs remains unclear. Little direct progress has been made towards vaccine development for humans; however, a great deal of work has been carried out to characterize certain enzymes shared by these fluke **(Cox *et al.*, 2005)**. Human and experimental animals develop a complex array of humoral and cellular immune responses during the course of infection **(Osman *et al.*, 1992; Shaker *et al.*, 1994)**. Both cellular and humoral immune responses were induced in the liver of cattle and buffaloes during infection with *F. gigantica* probably by antigens released by the developing flukes and by damage caused by the flukes during their migration in the liver **(Molina and Skerratt, 2005)**.

Most workers investigating the mechanisms of immunity of *Fasciola* have used the rat as their experimental animal because of its superior ability to develop resistance to reinfection. **Rajasekariah and Howell (1977)** showed that, previously infected rats resist an oral challenge, but develop no immunity to a similar challenge given intraperitonealy (i.p.). In contrast, **Kelly *et al.* (1980)** claimed that, acquired resistance is expressed as effectively against i.p. challenge against oral challenge. A recent observation suggests that at least two distinct mechanisms may be involved. Resistance at the intestinal barrier might be non-specific and thymus-independent, whereas specific acquired immunity operates beyond the intestine **(Smithers, 1982)**.

Several lines of evidence support the role of T cells in protective immunity. In vaccine trials with *F. hepatica*, antibody titers were not generally associated with protection **(Dalton *et al.*, 1996)**. Protection in *F. gigantica* vaccine trials were not antibody mediated **(Estuningsih *et al.*, 1997)**. Passive transfer of protective immunity required volumes of immune serum too large to be consistent with humoral based protection (**Armour and Dargie, 1974**). In contrast, lymphoid cells have proven to be more efficient at transferring immunity (**Armour and Dargie, 1974; Chapman and Mitchell, 1982b**). While the studies support a role for T cells, little work has been conducted characterizing specific T cell responses in *F. hepatica* infection. Better elucidation of host immunity is critical to the logical development of vaccines against *F. hepatica* and related trematodes. In previous work, **Shoda et al. (1999)** have characterized Th cell lines and $CD4^+$ T cell clones specific for *F. hepatica* soluble worm antigen (SWA). The T helper (Th) cell lines co-expressed the cytokines, interleukin-4 (IL-4), and interferon-gamma (IFN-γ); identifying these lines as having unrestricted T helper type 0 cell (Th0)-like phenotypes. Similarly, most T cell clones expressed a Th0-like cytokine profile; a few expressed an IL-4 dominant Th2–like profile, but no clones were identified with IFN-γ dominant Th1 type profile. Th2-like responses has also been implicated by the predominant immunoglobulin G1 (IgG1) response upon re-exposure of previously infected cattle (**Clery et al., 1996; Brown et al., 1999**). These IgG1-based responses are consistent with recent data on *Schistosoma*-infected human suggesting that Th2 responses are inversely related to disease in the natural host (**Mwatha et al., 1998**).

In the study of cattle fascioliasis, lymphocyte proliferation assays showed a positive correlation between the cumulative lymphocyte response to fluke antigen and the mature fluke burden. The antibody responses, moreover, was dominated by the IgG1 isotype. Lastly, blood cultures stimulated with adult fluke antigen failed to produce IFN-γ, a Th1–type cytokine, in keeping with previous work showing a low level if IFN-γ transcripts in *F. hepatica*-specific bovine Th-cell clones (**Brown et al., 1994**). In primary infected cattle, however, an early production of IFN-γ has been recorded (**Clery and Mulcahy, 1998**), suggesting differing immune response in chronically infected and naïve infected cattle. Recently, **Brown et al. (1999)** demonstrated that, most $CD4^+$T-clones co-express IFN-γ and IL-4, underscoring the heterogeneous nature of the cytokine response by $CD4^+$T-cells. Little is known about how the rate at which the infection is demonstrated affects the development of resistance.

During the migration of *F. hepatica* to the bile duct of the mammalian host, numerous antigens that are potentially capable of inducing a specific Th_2-like response are expressed (**Reddington et al., 1984**). Of particular interest is the tegument and outer glycocalyx, which are maintained through constitutive granule secretion by developmentally regulated secretory cells (**Shoda et al., 1999**). The antigenicity of the glycocalyx has been demonstrated by incubation of worms with immune sera which resulted in extensive Ig surface coating, although rapid turnover mediated by granule secretion apparently permitted antibody shedding (**Hanna, 1980**). Both rapid turnover and developmentally regulated expression of distinct secretory cells may contribute to immune evasion by the parasite (**Tkalcevic et al., 1996**). They have focused on tegument antigens that are common to the juvenile and adult worm stages as potential targets of the immune response directed against both life stages. One candidate protein is the 12 kDa *F. hepatica* thioredoxin molecules that has been previously identified by immunoscreening using *F. hepatica* immune sera and has been characterized as being present on both NEJs and adult worm stages (**Richardson, 1994**).

Increased levels of eosinophils are found in the lamina propria of the rat small intestine 3 wk PI with *F. hepatica* and there is a marked increase in intestinal Eosinophilia immediately after challenge (**Doy et al., 1978**). Adult flukes introduced into peritoneal cavity of immune rats show palliating attachment of cells, mostly Eo, around there tegument within 1.5 hr, other Eo degranulate at a distance from the parasite. The destruction of the fluke's tegument however, appears to be also affected by neutrophils and macrophages (**Bennett et al., 1980**).

Recently, some aspects of immune response against *F. hepatica* in the goat have been described, such as antibody production and lymphocyte proliferative response to excretory/secretory (E/S) products (**Martinez-Moreno et al., 1997**). But the nature of that responses and its relationship with the pathogenesis of the disease have not been considered. In sheep and rats, there are some work described how NEJs induce a granulomatous lesion in the hepatic parenchyma, with numerous macrophages, lymphocytes and Eo (**Chauvin and Boulard, 1996**). This reaction is dependent on cell-mediated responses against parasite, but no such studies have been carried out in goat fascioliasis.

By using peripheral blood mononuclear cells (PBMNCs), proliferation assays assess the cell mediated immune response involved in fascioliasis under the same experimental conditions. **Bossaert et al. (2000)** have paid a special attention to the type of cells involved in the immune response. Eo have been reported as the main leukocyte-type helping to fight parasitic infection (**Hansen et al., 1999**). In rats, Eo may have a role in the development of resistance to reinfection (**Davies and Goose, 1981; Milbourne and Howell, 1990**). In sheep, skin Eo counts following an intradermal reaction to mitogens appeared to correlate with the level of resistance to a *Trichostronglus colubriformis* infection (**Rothwel et al., 1991**). A possible involvement of Eo in antibody-dependant cell-mediated cytotoxicity (ADCC) mechanisms (**Burden et al., 1983; Van Milligen et al., 1998**) and in IgE-dependant hypersensitivity reaction was reported (**Doy et al., 1981**).

In vitro, **Doy and Hughes (1980)** had shown that, Eo from a mixed population of rat peritoneal cell selectively adhere to the tegument of *F. hepatica* NEJs in the presence of serum from previously infected rats. An artificially raised antiserum to dead fluke antigens failed to induce Eo adherence. Neutrophils and Eo from cattle were also shown to adhere in large numbers to

NEJs coated with antibody from infected cattle, attachment was dependent on fraction crystalline (Fc) receptor, although the adherence of Eo was more prolonged than that of the neutrophils. Despite this cell-parasite interaction, damage to the fluke was measured by chromium release could not be demonstrated, although it was subsequently shown that a major basic protein isolated from cattle Eo caused damage and death of NEJs **(Duffus and Frankes, 1980)**.

Th1, Th2, B cells and macrophages are all activated during *Fasciola* infection **(Osman and Abo El-Nazar, 1999)**. They cooperate in overcoming the parasite and work in benefit of the host. The immunological response is carefully regulated by the aid of a complex network of immunoregulatory mediators (cytokines) **(Khalil et al., 1999)**.

Interleukin-1 (IL-1) is well known as a pro-inflammatory macrophage/monocyte driven cytokine, secrete by B cells as well as other cell types. It achieves alone or with other cytokines namely tumor necrosis factor (TNF), IL-6 and IL–8, as a set of systematic events modulating the inflammatory reaction. It co-stimulates the cell activation and promotes B-cell maturation **(Chensue et al., 1993; Ruth et al., 1996)**. IL-4 is released predominantly by Th2 cells; it has important effects in relation to T and especially B cell function. It is primarily an anti-inflammatory cytokine that causes coordinate down-regulation of macrophage derived IL-1 and TNF. It has inhibitory effects on macrophage function. It provides a potent stimulus for B cell switching to production of IgE antibody. As such it is important from clinical point of view in relation to parasitic infections in which IgE antibody-mediated response plays an important role **(Medhat et al., 1998; Schof et al., 1998)**. IgE is present in the serum of healthy individuals at extremely low levels. Its level rises in response to parasitic infections. The induction of IgE synthesis by parasitic infection has been shown to be T cell dependent and these cells appears to exert their effect through the production of soluble factors that enhance the production of IgE by B cells. It activates mast cells and it is important in defense against parasitic infections, e.g. worms **(Yamaguchi et al., 1997)**.

- **Resistance to infection**

The relative susceptibility or resistance of the host to *Fasciola spp.* infection is associated with the biochemical characteristics of parasites and the host immune response during fascioliasis **(Spithill et al., 1999b; Meeusen and Piedrafita, 2003)**. Sheep are susceptible to *F. hepatica* infection but less susceptible to *F. gigantica* infection **(Boyce et al., 1987; Roberts et al., 1997)**.

Acquired resistance to a secondary *F. gigantica* infection following a primary infection or vaccination has been demonstrated in cattle, goats and sheep **(Haroun and Hillyer, 1986)**. Low or no resistance is seen hamsters and mice and the infection is highly pathologic in both the acute and chronic phases. In heavy infection death is the usual sequel **(Smithers and Doenhoff, 1982)**.

It is well established that sheep do not acquire resistance to *F. hepatica* as determined from the observed yields of mature parasites after primary and secondary infections with *F. hepatica* **(Haroun and Hillyer, 1986; Boyce et al., 1987)**. In European sheep, yields of *F. hepatica* ranged from 16 to 38 % and from 13 to 31 % after primary and secondary infection, respectively, indicating that resistance to *F. hepatica* does not develop in these sheep breeds **(Boyce et al., 1987)**. In contrast, acquired resistance to *F. gigantica* has been observed in sheep. **Flynn et al. (2007)** reported that, infection with *F. hepatica* results in polarization of the host's immune response and generation of Th2 immune responses, which are known to be inhibitory to Th1 responses.

Buffaloes were highly susceptible to *F. gigantica* infection, and this susceptibility could be associated with the late and weak cellular immune response in the early phase of infection **(Zhang et al., 2006)**. There was a trend toward higher parasite-specific IgG2 titers in sheep infected with lower worm burdens, suggesting that higher *F. gigantica* or *F. hepatica* burdens suppress IgG2 responses. The findings of this study suggested that, in early infection in a permissive host, *F. hepatica* appears to be more pathogenic than *F. gigantica* because of its rapid increase in size and the speed of its progression through the migratory phases of its life cycle **(Raadsma et al., 2007)**. **Cervi et al. (1999)** reported that, The E/S antigen of *F. hepatica* is involved in the suppressive phenomena of cellular immune responses in rats.

Most workers investigating the mechanism of immunity to *Fasciola h*ave used the rat as their experimental animal because of its superior ability to develop resistance to reinfection.

Smithers (1982) suggested that, resistance at the intestinal barrier might be non-specific and thymus-independent, whereas specific acquired immunity operates beyond the intestine. **Armour and Deargie (1974)** noted that, when high levels of immunity are transferred with serum, the worms of the challenge appear to be destroyed before they enter the liver. On the other hand, a similar level of protection against a challenge after adoptive transfer of cells is invariably accompanied by marked liver lesions associated with cellular infiltrates and dead immature parasites.

Bossaert et al. (2000) have paid special attention to the type of cells involved in the immune response. Eo have been reported as the main leukocyte-type helping to fight parasitic infection **(Butterworth, 1977)**. The cellular immune response to *F. hepatica* infection in different animal species has been widely studied. Especially, in *F. hepatica*-infected sheep, a significant transient proliferation *in vitro* of PBMNCs stimulated by parasite antigens appears during the first wk of infection **(Moreau et al., 1998; Mulcahy et al., 1999)**. PBMNCs proliferation induced by *F. gigantica* E/S products increased from 2 wk PI with a peak at 5 wk PI **(Zhang et al., 2006)**. Peripheral blood Eo counts increased as previously described in *F. hepatica* and in *F. gigantica* infected sheep **(Chauvin et al., 1995; Hansen et al., 1999; Zhang et al., 2005)**. Eo numbers increased significantly from 3 wk PI in *F. gigantica*-infected buffaloes and displayed a peak at 8 wk PI **(Zhang et al., 2006)**.

Neutrophils and Eo from cattle were also shown to adhere in large numbers to NEJs coated with antibody from infected cattle **(Duffus and Frankes, 1980)**. The total number of hepatic mononuclear cells increased significantly following infection, but the proportion of Natural killer (NK) cells did not change. After infection, these cells were found around the portal space, around the centrolobular vein, in the periportal fibrosis and in the band of collagen. However, no NK cells could be detected in or around the granuloma during infection **(Tliba et al., 2002)**.

The cell mediated immunity to *F. hepatica* antigens in cattle is investigated by establishing the lymphocyte proliferation and tests for quantitative determination of IL2 production **(Oldham and William, 1985)**. Some aspects of the immune response against *F. hepatica* in the goat have been described, such as antibody production and lymphocyte proliferative response to E/S products **(Martinez-Moreno et al., 1997)**. In sheep and rats, there are various data describing how the NEJs induce a granulomatous lesion in the hepatic parenchyma, depending on cell-mediated response against parasite with numerous macrophages, lymphocytes and Eo **(Chauvin and Boulard, 1996)**.

Bovine peripheral blood lymphocytes isolated 2-5 wk PI undergo strong proliferative responses upon co-culture with *F. hepatica* specific antigen, although this response is transient and lymphocytes gradually lose the ability to respond to *F. hepatica* antigens as the infection matures **(Clery and Mulcahy, 1998; McCole et al., 1999)**. The local cellular response may not, however, always reflect that found in the periphery: in mice and rats, both the specificity and isotype of antibody **(Meeusen and Brandon, 1994)**, together with PBMNCs cytokine profiles **(Tliba et al., 2002)** have been found to differ in the different body and immune compartments examined.

Waldvogel et al. (2004) investigated *F. hepatica* specific IL-4 and IFN-γ messenger ribonucleic acid (mRNA) expression in PBMNCs from calves experimentally infected with *F. hepatica*. Cells were collected prior to infection and on days 10, 28 and 70 PI. Interestingly, PBMNCs responded to stimulation with *F. hepatica* E/S products and expressed high amounts of IL-4 but not of IFN-γ mRNA suggesting that *F. hepatica* induced a Th2 biased early immune response which was not restricted to the site of infection. Later in infection, IL-4 mRNA expression decreased whereas IFN-γ mRNA expression increased slightly.

In vitro, it is established that the cytokine production of monocytes from patients with acute or chronic fascioliasis is increased **(Khalil *et al.*, 1999)**. IL-8 and IL-6 are produced in higher amounts from the monocytes of patients with acute fascioliasis compared to the healthy controls. The production of these lymphokins is decreased during the chronic stage of the disease in comparison to the acute stage of the disease.

The production of IL-1 from mononuclear phagocytes, IL-4 from Th2 lymphocytes and IgE level are measured in patients with fascioliasis during the acute and chronic stage of the disease and after triclabendazole (TCBZ) treatment **(Allam *et al.*, 2000)** The levels of IL-1 and IL-4 are significantly decreased and the IgE level is increased both in acute and chronic stage of fascioliasis. After the drug treatment, the cytokine values restore to the control.

Osman *et al.* (1989) reported that, antibodies, cytotoxic T-cells, activated macrophages, NK cells and many other cells, mediators of the ADCC, and modulator of the immune system as cytokines, are involved in the immune mechanisms, which are efficient against parasites.

Clery and Mulcahy (1998), established early stimulation of IFN-γ production in the peripheral lymphocytes of *F. hepatica* infected cattle. Others also established that the IFN-γ level was increased only during the first 2 wk PI the *F. hepatica* in sheep, IL-10 is secreted mainly during the first 6 wk PI and monocytes were inhibited till the 35th wk PI **(Moreau *et al.*, 1998)**.

3. Treatment

A number of drugs have been used to control fascioliasis in animals. Drugs differ in their efficacy, mode of action, price, and viability. Fasciolicides (drugs against *Fasciola spp.*) fall into five main chemical grs:

Halogenated phenols: bithionol (Bitin), hexachlorophene (Bilevon) and nitroxynil (Trodax).

Salicylanilides: closantel (Flukiver, Supaverm) and rafoxanide (Flukanide, Ranizole).

Benzimidazoles: triclabendazole (Fasinex), albendazol (Vermitan, Valbazen), mebendazol (Telmin) and luxabendazole (Fluxacur).

Sulphonamides: clorsulon (Ivomec Plus).

Phenoxyalkanes: diamphenetide (Coriban).

TCBZ is considered as the most common drug due to its high efficacy against adult as well as NEJ flukes. It is used in control of fascioliasis of livestock in many countries. Nevertheless, long-term veterinary use of TCBZ has caused appearance of resistance to *F. hepatica* in sheep **(Overend and Bowen, 1995)**.

The cost of the treatment with TCBZ prohibits its wide adoption by rural producers in developing countries. Scientists have started to work on the development of new drug. Recently, a new Fasciolicides was successfully tested in naturally and experimentally infected cattle in Mexico. This new drug is called compound Alpha and is chemically very much closed to TCBZ **(Ibarra et al., 2004)**.

Treatment is too late to decrease or avoid the side effects of the infection, also the extensive use of these drugs increase the risk of developing resistance to them. So, diagnosis is very important specifically early one to control the effect and spreading of infection.

4. Antigens-derived *Fasciola*

- Tegumental antigens (TA)

The tegument of *F. hepatica* provides the interface at which the host immune system interacts with the parasite. Its structure has been determined by microscopy to be a syncytium formed by the fusion of specialized tegumental cells located beneath the longitudinal and lateral muscle layers **(Bennett and Threadgold, 1975)**. It is speculated that protein expression in the tegument regulates and plays an important part in the fluke's defense against the host's immune system **(Bennett et al., 1980)**.

Three types of nucleated cells are found within the nucleated layer of the tegument, which are active during various stages of the fluke's development within the mammalian host **(Hanna, 1980)**.

Initially type o (To) bodies are produced but during the migratory stage, they are the first to become active and then only within the metacercariae and the NEJs stage. These cells are known to produce granules that are then released at the apical surface of the NEJs fluke allowing for the continual turnover of the outer tegument in response to host antibody attachment **(Hanna, 1980)** and there is a switch to type 1 (T1) bodies and on reaching the bile duct type 2 (T2) bodies become predominant **(Bennett and Threadgold, 1975)**.

- Somatic antigens

Somatic antigens were fractionated by column chromatography for diagnosis of human fascioliasis. Somatic extracts of adult *F. hepatica* have been used both as a vaccine to induce resistance to challenge and to monitor the host immune response to infection. **Sinclair and Joyner (1974)** reported a 54% decrease in the fluke burden following challenge with the worms extract when compared to untreated control rabbits.

The humoral response to adult somatic antigens has also been examined by indirect fluorescent antibody-labeling of plastic embedded sections of NEJs and adult flukes. Estimates of the levels of specific IgG and IgA antibodies in the serum and bile were determined during the course of infection **(Hughes et al., 1981)**.

The immune response of sheep to somatic components of adult *F. hepatica* was studied during an experimental infection. Antibodies against adult fluke somatic antigens were detected by thin layer immunoassay from the 2nd wk PI. Similarly, the results of western blotting (WB) analysis showed a specific recognition of several components as early as 2 wk PI. However, an increase in the number and intensity of bands with time of infection was observed in the patterns of antigenic recognition towards components of 20-23 kDa in the somatic preparation of *F. hepatica*, especially noticeable after the 6th wk PI. Since these polypeptides were recognized by all infected animals, they could play an important role in the diagnosis of sheep fascioliasis **(Ruiz-Navarrete et al., 1993)**. Somatic antigens of *F. gigantica, G. explanatum, S. spindale* and *hydatid* cyst ingredients were analyzed to identify the cross-reactive antigens among them using WB technique **(Yokananth et al., 2005)**.

- **Excretory/Secretory antigens (E/S)**

Several *F. gigantica* antigens with immunodiagnostic potential have been identified in preparations of the flukes and their E/S products. These E/S antigens are probably composed of molecules released from the continuous turnover of the glycocalyx coating the tegument surface membrane as well as some enzymes released from the caecum. E/S antigens contained several enzymes such as glutathione-S-transferase (GST), CP and CL **(Espino and Finaly, 1994)**. It was found that CP of *F. hepatica* is very important candidates for a vaccine antigen because of their role in fluke biology and in the host-parasite relationship **(Wedrychowicz et al., 2007)**.

Subproteomics has been used to compare E/S products produced by adult *F. hepatica in vivo*, within ovine host bile, with classical exhaust *in vitro* E/S methods. Only CL proteases from *F. hepatica* were identified in our ovine host bile preparations. Several host proteins were also identified including albumin and enolase with host trypsin inhibitor complex identified as a potential biomarker for *F. hepatica* infection. Time course *in vitro* analysis confirmed CL proteases as the major constituents of the *in vitro* E/S proteome. In addition, detoxification proteins, actin, and the glycolytic enzymes enolase and glyceraldehyde-3-phosphate dehydrogenase were all identified *in vitro*. WB of *in vitro* and *in vivo* E/S proteins showed only CL proteases were recognized by serum pooled from *F. hepatica*-infected animals. Other liver fluke proteins released during *in vitro* culture may be released into the host bile environment via natural shedding of the adult fluke tegument. These proteins may not have been detected during our *in vivo* analysis because of an increased bile turnover rate and may not be recognized by pooled liver fluke infection sera as they are only produced in adults. This study highlights the difficulties identifying authentic E/S proteins ex host, and further confirms the potential of the CL proteases as therapy candidates **(Morphew et al., 2007)**.

Serradell et al. (2007) observed that, E/S products induced an early apoptosis of rat peritoneal Eo and that this phenomenon was time- and concentration-dependent. Furthermore, activation of protein tyrosine kinases (TyrK) and caspases were necessary to mediate the Eo apoptosis induced by the E/S products, and that carbohydrate components present in these antigens were involved in this effect. They described for the first time the ability of E/S products from *F. hepatica* to modify the viability of Eo by apoptosis induction. Besides that, we have observed Eo apoptosis in the liver of rats 21 days after *F. hepatica* infection. The diminution in Eo survival in early infection could be a parasite strategy in order to prevent a host immune response.

Ortiz et al. (2000) used E/S, somatic and surface antigens of adult *F. hepatica* for antibody response determination in dairy cattle naturally infected with *F. hepatica*. They reported that, antibody responses were developed against 60-66 kDa in E/S and surface antigens and 17 kDa in somatic antigen. **Qureschi et al. (1995)** used E/S antigens and reported that, at approximately 15 kDa *F. hepatica* E/S antigens can be used for species specific diagnosis in cattle. **Hillyer and Soler De Galanes (1991)**, obtained sera from human patients, calves, sheep, and rabbits infected with *F. hepatica* and tested the WB techniques with *F. hepatica* E/S antigens in order to evaluate their immunodiagnostic potential. Researchers reported that the serum samples from humans, rabbits, cattle, and sheep infected with fascioliasis recognized two antigenic polypeptides of 17 and 63 kDa in the form of sharp bands.

The E/S antigens of *Fasciola spp.* or their partially purified components are the most common sources of antigens for use in ELISA methods and antibodies to these antigens can be detected as early as 2 wk and peak concentrations are reached at 8-10 wk PI **(Fagbemi and Guobadia, 1995)**.

Evaluation of efficacy of E/S antigen by ELISA **(Osman et al., 1995)** revealed that, the crude preparation had 100% sensitivity. 94% specificity and 98% accuracy at cut off level of 0.3 in acute cases and positive results in 77% of chronic cases. Cross reactivity with *Schistosoma* (*S.*) and *Toxoplasma* was reported. So E/S is recommended for diagnosis of fascioliasis in acute cases. However, low positive results with chronic case may limit its application in routine investigation adding to the cross reaction with sera of other parasites.

The E/S antigen of *F. gigantica* was tested by ELISA against sera from fascioliasis, schistosomiasis and hydatidosis cases to determine its sensitivity and specificity in the detection of specific IgG antibodies **(Ortiz et al., 2000)**. The sensitivity of E/S antigen was found to reach up to 100% and the specificity of E/S was 89.47% and 86.8% for IgG and IgM, respectively **(Mousa, 1994)**. Cattle naturally exposed to *F. hepatica*, in Cajamarac, Peru; develop a significant IgG response to this parasite E/S antigen **(Ortiz et al., 2000)**.

- The E/S products of adult *F. hepatica* released during the course of the infection have been investigated. **Cuperlovic and Movsesijan (1972)**, using a fluorescent antibody test, found the caecal contents of adult flukes gave the strongest specific fluorescence during the course of infection. Fluorescent labeling also occurred on the epithelial cells lining the uterus and excretory ducts as well as the spermatogenic cells. **Ericksen and Flagsted (1974)** proposed that, host resistance induced by subcutaneous (s.c) implantation of adult worms might be directed against the fluke's metabolic or E/S products. The finding of **Goose (1978)**, in which the E/S products of adults were found to be toxic to the lymphocytes from infected rats, suggested that some parasite products released many services to protect the parasite. E/S products have served as effective immunogens when mature flukes, contained within diffusion chambers, were implanted i.p. or s.c in rats. Resistance was imported by these implanted flukes whether they were present at the time of challenge or if they had been removed 2 wk earlier **(Haroun et al., 1980)**. **Proteases**

The ability of flukes to secrete proteolytic enzymes is critical for their survival in the definitive host, facilitating migration, and utilization of host tissue as nutrient and cleaving of host Igs **(Mulcahy and Dalton, 1998)**. A major component of the enzymes secreted by *F. gigantica* consists of cysteine proteases (CP), of which two major forms have been characterized, cathepsin L1 (CL1) and cathepsin L2 (CL2) **(Fagbemi and Hillyer, 1991&1992; Smith et al., 1993; Dowd et al., 1994)**.

Cells of the fluke gut produce these enzymes, which are homologous to mammalian lysosomal enzymes, CL1 and CL2 proteinases which act in the gut to breakdown ingested blood and other tissue, and are also regurgitated by the flukes. CL1 has been shown to cleave Igs in the hinge region and then prevent antibody-mediated attachment of Eo to NEJ flukes **(Carmona et al., 1993; Smith et al., 1993)**. The fluke CL1 and CL2 can also cleave host collagen and other extra cellular matrix proteins **(Beresain et al., 1997)**. Several reports have demonstrated that, proteases from parasites may be useful as protective vaccine **(Knox, 1994)**. It was found that, the secreted proteases were able to cleave Ig, a finding that strengthened the case for targeting these proteases as potential vaccine antigens for controlling infection with *F. gigantica* **(Chapman and Mitchell, 1982a)**. **Yamasaki and Aoki (1993), Heussler and Dobbelaere (1994) and Wijffels et al. (1994a)** revealed that, the secreted adult proteases are of the CL class.

CL of *Fasciola*, formulated in Freund's adjuvant, has been shown to protect cattle against *F. gigantica* **(Dalton et al., 1996)** and to induce high reduction (>70%) in the output of eggs by the parasites in vaccinated sheep **(Wijffels et al., 1994b)** and cattle **(Dalton et al., 1996)**. These results suggested a critical role for Freund's adjuvant in vaccine efficacy using CL that may relate to the induction of a certain arm of the immune responses.

- **Hemoglobin**

Another molecule isolated from *F. gigantica* secretion has been termed fluke hemoglobin (FHb), because it contains a hem gr and is likely to function in oxygen transport and was shown to have an absorption aspect similar to hemoglobin **(McGonigle and Dalton, 1995)**. From *F. gigantica,* a hem-containing protein was isolated and characterized from the E/S material of adult this protein has an apparent molecular weight (Mw) greater than 200 kDa. This molecule, used in combination with CL1 or CL2 seems also to be a useful vaccine antigen. CL2 and FHb, for example, produced reductions in fluke burden of 72% when administrated to cattle in Freund's adjuvant. Importantly, this combination also resulted in a 98% decrease in fecundity, perhaps due to a reduction in oxygen delivery by the hemoprotein. Egg shell production requires oxidative metabolism **(Bjorkman and Thorsell, 1963)**.

- **Proteases (Antigen)**

Structural fibrillar, α-helical and coiled-coil protein of approximately 100 kDa in the muscle and in some cases in the tegument, however some authors have shown the existence of extra muscular isoforms in larval stages of *S. japonica* **(Cancela *et al.*, 2004)**. It is widely distributed among invertebrates but absent in vertebrates. Also, it is considered as immunodominant antigen during infection caused by different flat worms such as *S. mansoni, Echinococcus granulosus, Taenia solium* (*T. solium*) and *F. gigantica* **(Lopez-Moreno *et al.*, 2003)**.

Antigen has also been used as a vaccine candidate against different parasitic disease, where different levels of response and protection have been achieved in animals **(Cancela *et al.*, 2004)**. In addition, Antigen from *T. solium* inhibits the classical pathway of complement through inhibition of C1 function **(Vazquez-Talavera *et al.*, 2001b)**. Immune response to Antigen induces Th2 type **(Jiz *et al.*, 2008)**. These findings suggest a multifunctional rule for the Antigen, not only as a structural component of contractile apparatus, but also a molecule capable of interacting with the host immune system in order to help parasite survival **(Cancela *et al.*, 2004)**.

Human T and B cell epitope mapping for Antigen of *T. Solium* was studied to indentify the immunologically relevant region of Antigen as a protective protein. Another study, in which characterization and protective potential of the immune response to *T. solium* Antigen was studied to give a protection against murine model of cysticercosis **(Vazquez-Talavera *et al.*, 2001a)**.

On the other hand, vaccination by peptides containing T cell epitopes from *S. mansoni* protein 14 (Sm 14), but not from Antigen, induces Th1 immune response that lead to reduction and partial protection against *S. mansoni* infection in mice **(Garcia *et al.*, 2008)**. Also, vaccination against fascioliasis by multivalent vaccine of stage-specific antigens, for example where

Cathepsin B (CB) and CL which are E/S materials from liver flukes and were used as target for vaccination. CB is predominant in juvenile stage of life cycle, while CL's are released throughout the cycle. They were used singly or in combination to vaccinate rats that were subsequently challenged with *F. hepatica* metacercariae leading to induction of immune response and yielded significantly fewer and small flukes than control gr **(Jayaraj *et al.*, 2009)**. Previous studies showed that immunization with recombinant Antigen from *Trichinella spiralis* (*T. spiralis*) (rTs-Antigen) formulated with Freund's adjuvant significantly reduced larval burden in mice after *T. spiralis* larval challenge. Since Freund's adjuvant is toxic and not a suitable adjuvant for clinical vaccine trials, we evaluated the ability of the adjuvants Montanide ISA206 and ISA720 to stimulate immune responses during rTs-Antigen immunization and to enhance protective immunity. The results revealed that immunization of BALB/c mice with rTs-Antigen formulated with either ISA206 or ISA720 triggered Th1 and Th2 immune responses similar to those produced by the conventional Freund's adjuvant formulation and also provided a similar level of protection against *T. spiralis* larval challenge. This indicates that the recombinant Ts-Antigen formulated with Montanide ISA206 or ISA720 may be an effective and safety vaccine strategy for trichinellosis **(Yang *et al.*, 2010)**.

The identification of the gene that encoding for Antigen of *Clonorchis sinensis* (CsAntigen) and characterized biochemical and immunological properties of its recombinant protein. CsAntigen showed a high level of sequence identity with Antigen from other helminths parasites. Recombinant CsAntigen (rCsAntigen) expressed in bacteria had an approximate molecular weight of 100 kDa and bound both human collagen and complement 9 (C9). The protein was constitutively expressed in various developmental stages of the parasite. Immunofluorescence analysis revealed that CsAntigen was mainly localized in the tegument, subtegumental muscles, and the muscle layer surrounding the intestine of the parasite. The rCsAntigen showed high levels of positive reactions (74.6%, 56/75) against sera from patients with clonorchiasis. Immunization of experimental rats with rCsAntigen evoked high levels of IgG production. These results collectively suggested that CsAntigen is a multifunctional protein that not only contributes to the muscle layer structure but also to non-muscular functions in host-parasite interactions. Successful induction of host IgG production also suggested that CsAntigen can be applied as a diagnostic antigen and/or vaccine candidate for clonorchiasis **(Park *et al.*, 2009)**.

The bovine lungworm *Dictyocaulus viviparus* Antigen (DvAntigen) was characterized on the transcriptional as well as genomic level. The identified genomic sequence comprises 19 introns compared to only 10 introns in the Caenorhabditis elegans orthologue. Quantitative real time PCR transcriptional analysis revealed Antigen transcription throughout the whole parasite's life cycle with the highest transcription rate in the agile moving first-stage larvae and the lowest in motionless hypobiosis induced third stage larvae. Recombinantly expressed DvAntigen was found to bind collagen and IgG. Thereby, this study showed that nematode Antigen has the capability for immunomodulation and thus may be involved in host immune defense **(Strube et al., 2009)**.

1. Diagnosis

However, *Fasciola* eggs may be found in the stools of uninfected patient who have eaten raw infected liver, leading to false positive diagnosis **(Bhamarapravati et al., 1983)**. The eggs found in the stool are very scarce and so concentration techniques are usually necessary **(Manson-Bahr and Apted, 1985)**. Furthermore, early diagnosis is not possible because eggs are not found in feces until flukes reach maturity, usually between 10-14 wk PI **(Armour et al., 1997)**.

During clinical and parasitological investigation, false negative results are common especially in light infections, leading to failure of diagnosis of many infected cases and to a strong underestimation of the prevalence of the disease **(De-Vias et al., 1992)**. For all of the disadvantages of the parasitological examination of fascioliasis, there was an approach to perform serological investigations. Various serological tests have been used for diagnosis. Almost all of these techniques concern the detection of circulating antibodies, and only a few are designed to detect circulating antigens and immune complexes **(Mas-Coma et al., 2005)**.

Early diagnosis is necessary for prompt treatment before irreparable damage to liver occurs **(Hillyer et al., 1992b)**. Diagnosis of fascioliasis, schistosomiasis and many other parasitic diseases in endemic areas depends mainly on the microscopic detection of eggs in the stool or urine (the parasitological diagnosis) **(Barreto et al., 1990)**, which is based on identification of eggs in stool, duodenal contents or bile, also by the recovery of adult worms during surgical exploration, after treatment or at autopsy. However, the eggs may be present in a very small number at irregular intervals, hence difficult to be found. Besides, the eggs may be transiently present in stool after ingestion of raw or undercooked liver from infected animals. The direct methods of diagnosing the eggs are usually unsatisfactory. The symptoms may be present for several wk before eggs are recovered in stool. Thus, the serologic tests are the alternative method of confirming early and extrabiliary human fascioliasis. However, cross-reactions with other helminthic antigen may confuse the interpretation of the results **(Haseeb et al., 2002)**. Thus prevention and control of the disease is important to provide a proper treatment before liver damage occurs. This will be achieved by early diagnosis of the disease and development of a proper vaccine for prophylaxis from infection **(Hillyer et al., 1992b)**.

The measurement of the hepatic enzymes gamma-glutamyl transpeptidase (γGT), aspartate aminotransferase (AST) and glutamate dehydrogenase (GLDH) in plasma merely indicates liver pathology and is not a specific test for fascioliasis **(Leclipteux et al., 1998)**. Eosinophilia is the most frequent laboratory abnormality. The computed tomography scan has become useful technique in the diagnostic work-up **(Hillyer, 1999)**.

Antibody-based serologic tests were used successfully to detect *F. hepatica* as early as 2-4 wk PI, an advantage over current sedimentation techniques, which do not detect worms before they mature and begin eggs shedding at approximately 8 wk PI. Several assays of immunoserological diagnosis of human fascioliasis, based on the detection of specific antibodies, have proved to be very useful. Such as the indirect Immunoflurescent assay (IIF) **(Deelder and Ploem, 1975)**, the enzyme-linked immunoelectrotransfer blot (EITB) **(Tsang et al., 1983)** and enzyme-linked Immunosorbant assay (ELISA) with its various modifications **(Osman et al., 1995; Maleewong et al., 1996)**.

Deelder and Ploem (1975) used IIF technique to diagnosis fascioliasis antibodies in human, rabbits and calves. The test proved to be one of the best tests, but the costs of an Immunoflurescent microscope, the subjectivity of reading the test, and the technical difficulties in evaluating large numbers of sera have hindered the wide application of IIF test **(Kagan, 1979)**.

Indirect hemagglutination test (IHA), was found to be more sensitive and specific for diagnosis of fascioliasis. It was indicated direct correlation between antibody titer and intensity of infection **(Hillyer and De-Ateca, 1979)**.

In counter immunoelectrophersis (CIEP), crude *Fasciola* antigens were used for detection of fascioliasis antibodies, but it showed a cross reactivity with sera of patients with schistosomiasis. However, when partially purified fractions of antigen were used, it reacted with fascioliasis patient sera only **(Mansour et al., 1983)**.

ELISA was evaluated by several investigators as a specific technique of high sensitivity for detection of human fascioliasis antibodies **(Khalil et al., 1990; Shaker et al., 1992)**.

Specific ELISA methods have been developed using adult fluke crude extracts E/S as antigens for the detection of serum antibodies **(Hassan et al., 1995; O'Neill et al., 1998)**. However, these assays showed limited specificity since *Fasciola* shares cross reactive antigens with antigens of many parasites, namely *Schistosoma* and *Echinococcus* **(Hassan et al., 1995)**. Specificity could be markedly improved by using proper anti-isotypes secondary antibodies. Unfortunately, information on the serum antibody isotype response in human is scarce **(O'Neill et al., 1998)**.

Serodiagnosis is generally performed by ELISA and WB methods using antigens derived from adult fluke extracts or E/S products **(Fagbemi and Guobadia, 1995; Clery et al., 1996; Sampaio-Silva et al., 1996)**. The E/S antigens of *Fasciola spp.* or their partially purified components are the most common source of antigens for use in ELISA methods and antibodies to these antigens can be detected as early as 2 wk and peak concentrations are reached at 8-10 wk PI **(Fagbemi and Guobadia, 1995)**.

The time course analysis of antibody response to *F. gigantica* infection in sheep was studied by ELISA and EITB. Sera from sheep experimentally infected with *F. gigantica* were reacted with E/S antigens of the worm before and after chemotherapy with oxyclozanide. In ELISA, there was a significant increase in anti-*Fasciola* antibody by 2 wk PI and there was a sharp decrease in antibody titer by 4 wk **(Guobadia and Fagbemi, 1995)**.

Used ELISA and micro-ELISA were used for serodiagnosis of fascioliasis employing E/S products from adult *F. hepatica*. The sensitivity of each method was 100% but the specificity was 100% for ELISA and 97% for micro-ELISA. The micro-ELISA could be used as a screening assay and ELISA could be used as a confirmatory method for serodiagnosis of fascioliasis **(Silvana et al. 2001)**.

Castro et al. (2000) investigated the dynamics of the appearance and persistence of antibodies using dot-ELISA after treatment of cattle naturally infected with *F. hepatica*. This is important in countries such as Uruguay, where the endemicity of cattle fascioliasis makes it necessary to distinguish antibodies from current and residual *F. hepatica* infection. ELISA with two CP of 26 kDa (Fas1) and 25 kDa (Fas2), obtained from the regurgitated material of adult worms, and were evaluated with serum samples from patients infected with *F. hepatica* and patients with other parasitic infections. The specificity of the ELISA was 98% for Fas1 and 100% for Fas2. ELISA with Fas2 is a highly sensitive and specific assay for immunodiagnosis of fascioliasis **(Córdova et al., 1999)**.

The use of CP from *F. hepatica* adult flukes for the serodiagnosis of sheep fascioliasis by the indirect ELISA test was studied. Two fractions from adult fluke homogenates, with apparent Mw of 28 and 34 kDa (P28 and P34 respectively), were characterized as CP. Both P28 and P34 fractions were electro eluted and used as antigens in two different indirect ELISA tests. Serum IgG level against P28 and P34 in goats infected experimentally with 200 metacercariae were determined and compared with those observed in an uninfected control gr **(Ruis et al., 2003)**.

ELISA tests using CP showed a rapid and consistent detection of specific IgG in all experimentally infected goats. The IgG response to P28 was the first to be detected as early as 2-3 wk PI and remained elevated throughout the experiment. The response to P34 was detected later (4-6 wk) and disappeared in some animals at 18 wk PI, while flukes were still present in the bile ducts. No significant differences were observed between the anti-P28 and anti-P34 IgG responses between animals receiving a primary or a challenge infection. The results of the study, although preliminary, were promising since the P28 ELISA was a reliable method for immunodiagnosis of *F. hepatica* infection in goats (**Ruis et al., 2003**).

A Glycoprotein (27 kDa) was isolated from crude somatic antigen of *F. gigantica* by two steps affinity chromatography and was used in early detection of experimental fascioliasis in cattle by indirect ELISA and in dot-ELISA formats, although, anti-27 kDa antibodies could be detected after 3 wk PI by dot-ELISA which was 1 wk later than indirect ELISA. Dot-ELISA was more convenient in field application. By dot-ELISA, the infection could be equally detected in animals infected with 100, 200 and 300 metacercariae of *F. gigantica* with high sensitivity (**Ghosh et al., 2005**).

Antigen detection also has advantage over antibody detection in that it implies current infection and as a parameter of active infection may increase the potential management of clinical disease (**Rodriguez-Osorio et al., 1998**). These antigens are shed by mature and late immature flukes in the bile duct, making early detection possible; and in detectable quantities (**Abdel-Rahman, 1996**), with an excellent potential for the sensitive and specific detection of the disease. In fact, serum from patients infected with *S. mansoni*, cysticercosis, hydatidosis and Chagas disease does not cross-react with the *F. hepatica*.

A *Fasciola* specific, 69 kDa antigen, probably similar to the 70 kDa reported by **Rodriguez-Osorio et al. (1998)**, was detected in sera from goat naturally infected with *F. hepatica*, this 69 kDa antigens has been identified using sera of infected sheep and E/S products of *F. gigantica* (**Guobadia and Fagbemi, 1996**).

Circulating E/S antigens have been detected in serum and feces of human, cattle, and rats, infected with *F. hepatica* using polyclonal antibody (pAb) and monoclonal antibody (mAb).

Clinically, human fascioliasis has to be differentially diagnosed from hepatic diseases as acute and chronic hepatitis, if the parasitological examination was unsatisfactory. So, ELISA for *F. hepatica* E/S antigens was evaluated in the immunodiagnosis of parasitologicaly proven cases of human fascioliasis. ELISA for *F. hepatica* E/S antigens gave 100% sensitivity and 100% specificity (**Haseeb et al., 2003**).

The 27-28 kDa E/S antigens partially purified from *F. gigantica* adult worms has been used as the sensitive and specific antigens for immunodiagnosis of human fascioliasis (**Tantrawatpan et al., 2003**). *F. hepatica* proteins (28 kDa) is one of diagnostic antigens in human fascioliasis without cross reaction with other human trematodiasis (**Kim et al., 2003**).

Adult somatic antigen extract of *F. gigantica* was compared with E/S antigens in ELISA for serodiagnosis of human fascioliasis. The absorbance values in ELISA using the adult somatic antigen were not significantly *(P>0.05)* different from the values obtained using E/S antigens. The diagnostic sensitivity, specificity and positive and negative predictive values (PPV and NPV) of the test using adult somatic extract as antigen were 100%, 98%, 70% and 100%, respectively. On the other hand, these values of the test using adult E/S antigens were 100%, 99.3%, 87.5% and 100%, respectively. It appears that, both somatic and E/S antigens are effective antigens for use in the serodiagnosis of human fascioliasis **(Maleewong *et al.*, 1996)**.

Rodriguez-Peréz and Hillyer (1995), described the detection of E/S antigens in sera of infected sheep by double antibody micro-ELISA. Numerous antigens are associated with the migrating fluke **(Qureschi *et al.*, 1995)**. However, the antigenic pattern changes quickly PI **(Tkalcevic *et al.*, 1996)**. Antigens of somatic origin or of E/S products can be detected as early as 4-6 wk PI **(Rodriguez-Peréz and Hillyer, 1995)**. The method has some disadvantages; immunocomplex formation tends to reduce the number of epitopes available for the test, thus, decreases the sensitivity **(Langley and Hillyer, 1989)**. Once the flukes enter the bile duct, their various antigenic products may no longer be circulating **(Hanna, 1980)** and because these tests require serum, testing of large herds can be difficult.

A simple and dot-ELISA techniques based on the specific rabbit anti-serum was 100% specific when tested using sera from nine cattle infected with *F. gigantica* and 27 uninfected cattle. A specific rabbit anti-serum and WB analysis were used to demonstrate the presence of highly reactive antigens of 26-28 kDa not only in an extract of adult *F. gigantica* but also in E/S products of the worms, in bile secretion and in the sera of cattle that were naturally infected with parasites **(Attallah *et al.*, 2002)**.

The antibody response and circulating antigen levels in bovine calves, experimentally infected with *F. gigantica*, were monitored using EITB and sandwich ELISA, respectively. When EITB was used, the infected calves' sera recognized the polypeptides in the range of 54-58 kDa as early as 2 wk PI. By 12th wk PI, the lower two polypeptides of 12 and 8 kDa had disappeared. In sandwich ELISA, the circulating 54 kDa and whole worm antigens of *F. gigantica* were detected in serum samples of infected calves as early as 2 wk PI and persisted until the end of experiment (26th wk PI). The 54 kDa antigen of *F. gigantica* appears to be specific and possesses promising immunodiagnostic potential for early prepatent diagnosis of bovine fascioliasis **(Velusamy *et al.*, 2004)**.

Materials and Methods

Rabbits

Newzealand white male rabbits, weighting approximately 1.5 Kg and about 1.5 months of age, were examined before the experiments (free from *Fasciola* and other parasitic infection), and maintained at the Schistosome biological supply program, Theodor Bilharz Research Institute, Giza, Egypt (SBSP/TBRI). They were kept under standard laboratory care (at 21°C, 45-55% humidity), and supplied with filtered drinking water ad libitum, 24% protein and 4% fat diet. Animal experiments have been carried out according to the internationally valid guidelines and ethical conditions **(Nessim *et al.*, 2000).**

1. Worms

Adult *F. gigantica* worms were obtained from the bile ducts and gall bladders of cattle livers naturally infected with parasite at a local slaughter house. The flukes were washed three to four times with phosphate buffered saline (PBS), pH 7.4, at room temperature to remove all traces of blood, bile and contaminating microorganisms **(Maggioli *et al.*, 2004).**

Metacercariae of *F. gigantica* were purchased from the SBSP-TBRI. Metacercariae were collected immediately in cellophane sheets after shedding from *Lymnaea natalensis* snails, and then gently removed by scrapping them off with two small glass plates and used for infection.

Worms and blood were collected randomly from naturally infected cattle's during several visits to local abattoir (75 animals infected by *Fasciola* worms and 30 healthy control animals). Blood samples were collected during slaughtering. The livers and gall bladders of animals were checked for the adult flukes. Sera were prepared in 0.1ml/aliquot, heat-inactivated and stored at -20°C until used.

2. Antigen Preparation and Purification

Adult clean *F. gigantica* worms were homogenized in 2 volume (vol.) of 20mM Tris-HCl buffer (BDH Chemicals, England) containing 5mM Phenylmethylsulfonyl fluoride (PMSF) as a protease inhibitor (Sigma–Aldrich, Louis, USA) at 20.000 rpm using IKA T20 homogenizer (IKA, Staufen, Germany). The homogenate was centrifuged at 30.000 rpm for 30 min. The entire process of homogenization and centrifugation was performed at 4°C. The supernatant fractions were decanted and assayed for protein content and stored at -20°C until used as crude extracts.

A. DEAE-Sephadex G-25 and G-200 ion exchange chromatography

Sephadex G-25 powder (Amersham Bioscience, Uppsala, Sweden) was swelled in about 300 ml of 0.5 M Tris-HCl buffer (pH. 7). Sephadex G-25 powder (5 gm) was added slowly to the buffer with gently stirring using glass rod, complete swelling takes 1-2 days at room temperature or 2 hours (hr), at 100°C, over boiling water. Swelling at high temperature also serves to deaerate the medium. Vigorous stirring, was avoided in order not to damage the particles. Five gm Sephadex G-25 powder were swelled to 22 ml beads.

After swelling of the DEAE-Sephadex, the initial supernatant was removed and washed extensively with 10mM Tris-HCl buffer (pH 6.5). Then slurry with 75% settled medium (swelled beads) to 25% buffer was prepared. The slurry was poured into 30 x 2.5 cm column (Bio-Rad) in one continuous motion down a glass rod held against the wall of the column; this step minimized the introduction of air bubbles. Following the settling of beads (G-25 and G-200) in the column, the column was equilibrated with 3 bed vol. (10mM Tris-HCl) and the approximate column binding capacity was determined. The sample was dialyzed versus the eluting buffer and its protein content was calculated. The outlet tubing of the column was then closed. The protein content ≤10% of column bed capacity was applied to the column using Pasteur pipette. The outlet was then opened and the beads were washed by 4 bed vol. eluting buffer. The substance of interest, Antigen is washed out of the gel and not adsorbed under these conditions **(Timanova et al., 1999)**. One ml fractions collected under gravity after G-25 ion exchange chromatography purification the target fraction (tubes with max. O.D readings were pooled and the pool) was run for more purification on G-200 ion exchange chromatography and absorbance at 280 nm of each fraction was measured. The specific fractions were then analyzed for final max. purification by sodium dodecyl sulphate polyacrylamide gel electrophoresis (SDS-PAGE), then protein content was colormetrically determined by the dye binding protein assay **(Bradford, 1976)** using commercially available BIO-RAD kits (BIO-RAD laboratories, Richmond, CA, USA).

B. Sodium dodecyl-sulfate polyacrylamide gel electrophoresis (SDS-PAGE)

In electrophoresis, the migration of proteins is dependent on the charge, size and shape of the molecules. However, in the presence of SDS, all proteins become negatively charged owing to their binding to negatively charged detergent molecules. When these SDS coated proteins are placed in an electric field, the separation of the proteins will depend only on their size and shape **(Laemmli, 1970)**. This criterium was used in detection and purification of Antigen.

Separating gel (12% acrylamide gel) was prepared by mixing 4 ml of stock acrylamide with 3.35 ml dist. H_2O, 2.5ml of 1.5M Tris-HCl, pH 8.8, 100µl 10% SDS (Merck, Damstadt, Germany), 50µl 10% APS (Sigma) and 5µl TEMED (Merck).

12% gel (1mm) was prepared under reducing condition according to Bio-Rad Lab. Model 595, Richmond, CA, USA manufacture and left to polymerize for 30-60 min. The top of the gel was covered with stacking gel. A plastic comb (1mm) was inserted into the large pore gel to form the sample wells and left to polymerize for 30 min. The comb was removed gently from the casting stand, mini-protein 1 multi casting chamber (Bio-Rad) and the slab cassette was placed in the inner cooling core of a mini-protein II cell (Bio-Rad). Electrode buffer (25 mm Tris, 192 mM glycine, 15 SDS), pH 8.3 was put in the upper and lower chamber.

Samples were prepared as 5μg of *F. gigantica* Antigen/ml. Sample buffer 1:4 (v/v) (4ml dist. H_2O, 1ml 0.5 M Tris-Hcl, pH 6.8, 0.8 ml glycerol, 1.6 ml 10% SDS) and 0.4 ml 0.05% (w/v) bromophenol blue (Koch-Light Lab. Coimbrook berk, England), and 0.4 ml β-mercaptethanol (Fluka, AG, Buchs, Germany) was prepared. Low M.w. kit standard protein (Bio-Rad) from 97 kDa was diluted in sample buffer 1:20 (v/v). The prepared samples and low M.w. standard were applied into the wells of the prepared gel (20 μl/well for sample and 10 μl for standard).

The current was connected by power supply 0-200 V DC (Behringwerke AG, Marbug-Lahn, Germany) and was turned on with the anode at the bottom. The run was started by 10 mA until the samples entered the stacking gel, and then the current was raised to 50 mA. The electrophoretic run is terminated after the bromophenol blue in the samples reaches the bottom of the gel.

After electrophoresis, the gel was stained in 0.1% Comassie blue (w/v) in methanol, acetic acid and water as 4:1:5 (v/v/v) for 2-4 hr, then the excess dye was removed from the gel by distaining solution to visualize the protein bands. After distaining the gel was stored in 5% acetic acid.

3. Reactivity and Specificity of *F. gigantica* Antigen

ELISA test involves the passive adsorption of antigen onto the surface of solid phase e.g. microtiter plate followed by addition of serum containing specific antibodies which may be labeled with an enzyme (conjugated anti-species Igs) (indirect ELISA). Indirect method can also be used by incubation of the coated antigen with unlabeled antibodies (primary) then enzyme labeled antibodies specific to the primary one. When a suitable substrate is added, hydrolysis occurs, the degree of which is proportional to the amount of attached enzyme. The enzyme and the substrate are chosen to produce colored enzyme-substrate breakdown.

Wells of polystyrene microtitre plates (96-flate bottomed wells, M129 A Dynatech) were coated with 100μl/well of *F. gigantica* Antigen at a concentration of 30ug/ml in 0.06M carbonate buffer, pH 7.4, then blocked with 200μl/well of 0.1% BSA (Sigma) in 0.1 M PBS, pH 7.4 for 1 hr at 37°C. The plates were washed with washing buffer (0.1 M PBS/T, pH 7.4) 5 times. Hundred μl of the Polyclonal antibodies against Antigen serially diluted (1/50, 100, 200, 400, 800, 1600) in 10% PBS were added to each well and incubated for 1 hr at 37°C. The plates were washed 3 times with washing buffer. Hundred μl of anti-rabbit IgG peroxidase conjugate (Sigma) diluted in 10% PBS (1/1000) were dispensed into each well and the plates were incubated for 1hr at 37°C. The plates were washed 5 times with washing buffer. Hundred µl of substrate solution dissolved in 25ml of 0.05 M phosphate citrate buffer pH 5 with peroxidase H_2O_2 (Sigma) were added to each well and the plates were placed in the dark at room temperature for 30 min. Fifty ml/well of 8N H_2SO_4 was added to stop the enzyme substrate solution. The absorbance was measured at 492 nm using ELISA reader (Bio-Rad microplate reader, Richomond, Ca).

4. Polyclonal antibodies Preparation

Rabbit anti-*Fasciola* serum was obtained by immunizing New Zealand white rabbits with *F. gigantica* Antigen. One mg of *F. gigantica* Antigen was given to each rabbit in the entire course of immunization. The rabbits received i.m. 1^{ry} dose injection at four sites of the femoral muscle [1 mg *F. gigantica* antigen mixed 1:1 in complete freund adjuvant (CFA) (Sigma)].

Two booster doses were given, each was 0.5 mg antigen emulsified in incomplete freund adjuvant (IFA). The subsequent boosting doses were given at 1 wk intervals after the 1^{ry} injection.

Blood samples were obtained from ear pinna of immunized rabbits before each immunizing dose and the titer was measured by indirect ELISA. At the end of the boosting doses, the rabbits were sacrificed, and the sera were collected, aliquoted and kept at -20°C.

Rabbit IgG purification steps were based on two different methods, Ammonium sulphate precipitation method and Caprylic acid purification method.

Proteins in solutions form hydrogen bonds with water through their exposed polar and ionic grs. When high concentration of highly charged ions such as ammonium sulfate is added, these grs compete with the proteins for binding to water. This removes the water molecules from the proteins and decreases its solubility, resulting in precipitation **(Nowotny, 1979).**

Saturated ammonium sulfate solution (SAS) (Sigma) was prepared by dissolving 100 gm of pure ammonium sulfate salt in 100 ml of dist. H_2O at 50°C and kept overnight at room temperature. After complete dissolving, the supernatant was separated and the pH was adjusted to be 7-7.2 by drops of concentrated ammonia.

SAS was added dropwise to rabbit anti-*Fasciola* serum to reach 50% saturation, with continuous stirring and then centrifuged for 20 min. at 12000 rpm in cooling centrifuge (Heraues) at 4°C. The supernatant was discarded, and then ammonium sulfate precipitation steps were repeated several times. The final precipitate was dissolved in a suitable amount of 0.01 M PBS. The ammonium sulfate was removed by dialysis against 0.01 M PBS, pH 7.2 for 72 days at 4°C.

The serum was dialyzed versus 3 mM Na acetate buffer, pH 4.8. Seven % caprylic acid was added drop wise with slow magnetic stirring for 30 min. at 4°C followed by centrifugation at 3000 rpm for 30 min. Albumin and other non-IgG proteins were separated and removed in the precipitate, While, the supernatant contained nearly pure IgG. the purity of the produced IgG was identified by SDS-PAGE **(Laemmli, 1970),** as described before

5. Periodate Method

Five mg of HRP (Sigma) was suspended in 1.2 ml of dist. H_2o. Then, 0.3 ml of freshly prepared sodium periodate was added and incubated at room temperature for 20 min. The HRP solution was dialyzed overnight against 1 mM sodium acetate buffer, pH 4 at 4°C with several changes of buffer solution. After preparation of pAb solution (5 mg/ml in 0.02M carbonate buffer, pH 9.6), the HRP was removed from dialysis tubing and was added to this solution. The mixture was left to incubate at room temperature for 2 hr.

Hundred µl of sodium borohydride was added and the solution was incubated at 4°C for 2 hr. The HRP-antibody conjugate was dialyzed with several changes against 0.01 M PBS, pH 7.2 **(Tijssen and Kurstak, 1984).**

6. Reactivity and Specificity of pAb Against *F. gigantica* Antigen

Wells of polystyrene microtitre plates (96-flate bottomed wells, M129 A Dynatech) were coated with 100µl/well of *F. gigantica* Antigen at a concentration of 30ug/ml in 0.06M carbonate buffer, pH 7.4, then blocked with 200µl/well of 0.1% BSA (Sigma) in 0.1 M PBS, pH 7.4 for 1 hr at 37°C. The plates were washed with washing buffer (0.1 M PBS/T, pH 7.4) 5 times. Hundred µl of the pAb against Antigen serially diluted (1/50, 100, 200, 400, 800 and 1600) in 10% PBS was added to each well and incubated for 1 hr at 37°C. The plates were washed 3 times with washing buffer. Hundred µl/well of anti-rabbit IgG peroxidase conjugate (Sigma) diluted in 10% PBS (1/1000) was dispensed and the plates were incubated for 1hr at 37°C. The plates were washed 5 times with washing buffer. Hundred µl/well of substrate solution dissolved in 25ml of 0.05 M phosphate citrate buffer pH 5 with peroxidase H_2O_2 (Sigma) were added and the plates were placed in the dark at room temperature for 30 min. Fifty ml/well of 8N H_2SO_4 was added to stop the enzyme substrate solution. The absorbance was measured at 492 nm using ELISA reader (Bio-Rad microplate reader, Richomond, Ca).

7. Standardization of Sandwich ELISA

The microtiter plates were coated with 100µl/well of purified IgG pAb with different concentrations (2.5, 5, 10, 20 and 40µg/ml) diluted in 0.06 M carbonate buffer, pH 9.6 and incubated overnight at room temperature. The plates were washed 3 times with washing buffer (0.1 M PBS/T, pH 7.4).

The free sites of the wells were blocked with 200µl/well of 1% BSA for 2 hr and incubated at 37°C. The plates were washed thrice with washing buffer. Hundred µl/well of *Fasciola* Antigen as positive control; 100µl/well of pooled positive or negative sera were added, and incubated for 2 hr at 37°C. The plates were washed 5 times, with washing buffer.

Then, 100µl/well of peroxidase-conjugated IgG pAb with different concentrations (5, 10, 25, 50 and 100µg/ml) was added to the wells, and incubated for 1 hr at room temperature. The plates were washed 5 times with washing buffer, 100µl/well of substrate solution [one tablet of O-phenylenediamine (OPD) dissolved in 25 ml of 0.05 M phosphate citrate buffer, pH 5 with urea hydrogen peroxidase] was added and the plates were incubated in the dark at room temperature for 30 min., 100µl/well of 8 N H_2SO_4 was added to stop the enzyme substrate reaction. The absorbance was measured at 492 nm using ELISA reader (Bio-Red microplate reader Richmond, Ca).

8. Parasitological Examination

The cellophane strips (20x30 mm) were kept soaked in the glycerin-malachite green mixture (100 ml pure glycerin, 100 ml dist. H_2o and 1 ml of 3% aqueous malachite green) for at least 24 hr. Approximately 1-2 g of stool sample was put on a disposable paper sheet and pressed with the sieve. A piece of sieved stool as transferred to fill the hole on the stainless steel template, then the template was put over a clean glass slide. The fecal sample was covered with a cellophane cover strip then the preparation was inverted and pressed down. The smear was allowed to stand for 24 hr. The entire preparation was examined under low power of microscope. The mean total number of eggs found on the 3 slides (each 50 mg feces) was multiplied by 20 to calculate the number of eggs/g stool (epg) **(Engels et al., 1997)**.

9. Immunodiagnosis of Sera

Seventy five samples of naturally infected cattle with *F. gigantica* and 30 healthy uninfected control samples were tested using sandwich ELISA and was compared with other parasites such as 30 samples infected with *S. mansoni*, *hydatid* and hookworm. All these animals' samples were collected after detection of adult worms in the dissected liver of naturally infected cattle's during several visits to local abattoir. Sensitivity and specificity of ELISA were evaluated.

10. Protection Strategy

16 Rabbits were divided into four grs of four rabbits each: Uninfected control gr, Infected control gr; rabbits were infected orally with 25 *F. gigantica* metacercariae, Immunized gr; rabbits were immunized with 1 mg of Antigen i.m. with equal vol. of CFA as 1^{ry} immunization on day 0. Booster doses, 1 ml of 0.5 mg Antigen mixed with an equal vol. of IFA, were administered after 2, 3 and 4 wk after the initial dose as 2nd, 3rd and 4th immunizations, Infected immunized gr; rabbits were immunized by the same regimen as gr C. Two wk after the 4th immunization, each of these animals was challenged orally with 25 *F. gigantica* metacercariae **(Muro et al., 1997)**. Blood samples were collected weekly from all grs during

the immunization schedule and every 2 wk after challenge infection from grs C and D till 12 wk PI.

11. Measurment of anti-*Fasciola* immunoglobulins

Anti-*Fasciola* IgM, total IgG and its isotypes IgG1, IgG2 and IgG4 subclasses were measured using of *Fasciola* Antigen by indirect ELISA. Wells of microtiter plates (Costar, Cambridge, MA) were coated with suspension of 5 µg of *Fasciola* Antigen (100µl/well) in binding buffer (0.05 M carbonate buffer, pH 9.6). The plates were covered and kept overnight at room temperature, then blocked with 1% BSA in PBS/T, pH 7.2 for 2 hr at room temperature. The plates were washed thrice with PBS/T and incubated with serum (100 µl/well), diluted 1:100 and 1:200 with 10% PBS for measurement of IgM, total IgG and its isotypes IgG1, IgG2 and IgG4, respectively, 1 hr in a water bath at 37°C, then washed thrice with PBS/T. Anti-human IgG peroxidase-labeled conjugate, gamma chain-specific (Sigma) and goat specific conjugate anti-human IgG4 (subclass-specific binding) labeled HRP (Sigma) were used at a dilution of 1:400 and 1:1000, respectively. Then plates were incubated for 30 min in a water bath at 37°C and washed 5 times with PBS/T and incubated with 100 µl/well of OPD Hcl substrate for 30 min. The reaction was stopped with 50 µl/well of 8 N H_2SO_4 and absorbance was measured as OD at 492 nm using a microplate ELISA reader (Bio–Rad microplate reader, Richmond, CA, USA). The cut off value was calculated as the mean OD of the uninfected control sera +2SD. Samples showing OD values equal to or greater than the cut off value were considered positive, and the samples showing OD lower than the cut off value were considered negative.

Cytokine profile

Briefly, 96-well microtiter plates (Nunc, Roskilde, Denmark) were coated with capture antibodies 100 µl of serum sample or recombinant cytokine. Following addition of the biotinylated detection antibody and streptavidin-alkaline phosphatase conjugate, the reaction was developed with para-nitrophenyl phosphate (Sigma). Absorbance at 405 nm was measured with a Benchmark reader (Bio-Rad laboratories Inc., Hercules, Calif.). Assays were performed in duplicate. The cytokine concentration was obtained from a regression curve prepared with the help of the Microplate Manager Software (Bio-Rad).

12. Statistics

It was carried out using one-way analysis of variance (ANOVA) according to **Campbell (1989)**. Comparison between 2 grs was done by the Student's t-test. The data were considered significant if *P<0.05*, highly significant if *P<0.01* and very highly significant if *P<0.001*. Percent reduction (PR) in all parameters was calculated according to **Fonseca *et al.* (2004)**.

Results

Purification and Characterization of Antigen From Adult *F. gigantica* Worms

The OD_{280} profile of the adult *F. gigantica* worm Antigen fractions obtained following purification of whole *F. gigantica* worm homogenate by DEAE Sephadex G-25 ion exchange chromatography. The eluted Antigen could be represented by fractions (no. 6-14) with a single peak with maximum OD value equal to 2.903 at fraction number 12. Fractions contained Antigen (no. 6-14) was further purified by DEAE-Sephadex G-200 ion exchange chromatography. One peak was obtained representing the column elution volume fractions which contain Antigen with OD value 2.420 at fraction number 8. The eluted protein fraction (no. 8) resulted from the different purification methods was analyzed by 12% SDS-PAGE under reducing conditions showing only one band at 97 kDa which represented Antigen. The whole worm homogenate obtained from adult *Fasciola* worms contains 8 mg/ml of total protein as measured by Bio-Rad protein assay, while, it was 4.9 mg/ml after primary purification with DEAE-Sephadex G-25 ion exchange chromatography and 2.6 mg/ml following secondary purification by DEAE-Sephadex G-200 ion exchange chromatography.

Reactivity of target antigen

The antigenicity of the purified target Antigen was tested by indirect ELISA technique. Serum samples from animals infected with *F. gigantica* gave strong reactivity against *Fasciola* Antigen with mean OD reading equal to 1.317 and very weak cross reactions were recorded with sera from animals infected with other parasites e.g., *S. mansoni*, *hydatid* and hookworm.

Reactivity of pAb against *F. gigantica* Antigen

Test blood samples were withdrawn from New Zealand white rabbits before and after the injection of each immunizing dose (4 samples). They were tested for the presence of uninfected specific anti-*Fasciola* antibodies by indirect ELISA (OD=0.310). An increasing antibody level started 1 wk after the 1^{ry} injection (OD=0.731), 1 wk after the 1st booster dose the titer reached (OD=1.91). Finally, three days after the 2nd booster dose, immune sera recorded a highest titer against *Fasciola* Antigen with OD reading of 2.97 at 1/250 dilution

Specificity of polyclonal antibody against *F. gigantica* Antigen

Reactivity of anti-*Fasciola* pAb against *Fasciola* Antigen and other parasite antigens (*S. mansoni*, hookworm and *hydatid*) was assayed by indirect ELISA to determine the specificity of Antigen. The produced anti-*Fasciola* pAb diluted 1/250 showed a strong reactivity to *Fasciola* Antigen. The mean OD reading at 492 nm for *Fasciola* was 2.660 compared to only 0.372, 0.316 and 0.362 for *S. mansoni*, *hydatid* and hookworm, respectively.

Rabbit anti-*F. gigantica* antibodies

The IgG-containing fraction of rabbit anti-*Fasciola* pAb was purified using different purification steps including ammonium sulfate precipitation followed by 7% caprylic acid precipitation method. The total protein content of crude immunized rabbit serum was 12.5 mg/ml. The yield of purification following each step was determined by the assessment of protein content. By using the 50% ammonium sulfate precipitation method, the protein content of pAb containing serum was decreased to 6.1 mg/ml, while following 7% caprylic acid precipitation, the content dropped to be only 3.2 mg/ml. The purity of IgG pAb after each purification step was assayed by 12% SDS-PAGE under reducing conditions. The purified IgG pAb was represented by L- and H-chain bands at 31 and 53 kDa, respectively. The pAb appears free from other proteins.

Sandwich ELISA Standardization

The anti-*F. gigantica* IgG pAb used for detection of *Fasciola* Antigen was employed as antigen capture and HRP pAb as conjugate in sandwich ELISA. The sandwich ELISA technique used for detection of *Fasciola* Antigen was previously demonstrated in the materials and methods, but it was necessary to do some preliminary standardization and optimization work first before the application of the technique on naturally infected animals' sera. The application of anti-*Fasciola* IgG pAb as antigen capturing antibody was evaluated by coating an ELISA plate with various concentrations of purified anti-*Fasciola* IgG pAb (2.5, 5, 10, 20 and 40μg/ml) in 0.01M carbonate coating buffer. The test was performed using one concentration of *Fasciola* Antigen (10μg/ml). Different concentrations of HRP conjugated rabbit anti-*Fasciola* IgG pAb (5, 10, 25, 50 and 100μg/ml) were evaluated.

It was found that, the optimum concentrations of coating and conjugate of pAb were 10μg/ml and 25μg/ml, respectively, against *F. gigantica* Antigen. Chosen concentrations were determined after subtraction of the background readings. Both concentrations were chosen as working dilutions for subsequent assays.

Parasitological examination

According to medical examinations during slaughtering, 75 animals were positive for *Fasciola* worms. But according to stool analysis by MIFC method and Kato Katz quantitative technique, only 50 animals (66.66%) were true positive and the rest of animals gave false negative results (25 animal, 33.33%). The intensity of infection was estimated as the number of ova/3 slides of stool, and calculated in gm/stool. According to the intensity of infection, animals were classified into two subgrs: Light infection: included 17 animals with the number of ova/3 slides of stool ranging from 9-40 ova with mean of 25±15.98. Heavy infection: included 33 animals with ova count more than 40 with mean of 64±18.30.

Immunodiagnosis of different sera samples

The data of *Fasciola* Antigen detection in the samples of the different studied grs. The cut off values for positivity was calculated as mean of uninfected control±2 SD and equaled 0.312. The OD values of *Fasciola* infected animals gr (1.76±0.406) was significantly higher $(P<0.001)$ than both of the uninfected control gr (0.198±0.098) and other parasite-infected grs. Seventy three cases were detected as positive samples of *F. gigantica* infected animals from 75 cases. These 2 samples were among the light infection subgr and the sensitivity of the assay was 97.33%. All of the 30 negative controls were below the cut off value; while, the data of 3 out of 30 other parasites-infected grs were above the cut off value giving 95% specificity.

Protection Protocol

Mean number of total worm burden and egg count

The mean total number of worm burden in grs of rabbits infected with 25 metacercariae of *F. gigantica* was 12±1.1. Immunization of infected rabbits with Antigen (gr D) stimulated a very highly significant $(P<0.001)$ decrease (5±1.3) in mean total number of worm burden with PR of 58.40%. When Antigen immunized rabbits were infected with 25 metacercariae (gr D), the mean total number of *F. gigantica* egg load was recorded (3255±145), showing a very highly significant decrease $(P<0.001)$ than infected control (gr B) (8440±213) with PR of 61.40%.

IgM and total IgG levels and its isotypes

Levels of IgM, IgG and isotypes (IgG1, IgG2 and IgG4) of anti-Antigen injected in normal and infected rabbits were assayed using indirect ELISA. The data showed an expected increase in IgM level in infected control (gr B) (0.71± 0.12) in comparison to normal control (gr A) (0.29±0.02). Immunization of rabbits with antigen (gr C) stimulated an elevation of IgM level (0.83±0.14) in comparison to its normal level with a very high significancy $(P<0.001)$.

After infection of preimmunized grs, IgM level was raised again. Rabbits immunized with Antigen before infection (gr D) recorded a significant $(P<0.05)$ level increase (0.96±0.12), which was higher than that of infected control level (gr B).

Infection itself causes an evident increase in the level of total IgG (1.14±0.12) (gr B) when compared to normal uninfected control rabbits (gr A) (0.24±0.03). The data revealed that, immunization of purified Antigen before infection (Gr C) have an extraordinary significant $(P<0.001)$ effect on total IgG, increasing its level higher than that of normal uninfected control gr (1.09±0.07). On the other hand, immunization with Antigen preinfection increases the IgG level in serum (1.55±0.13).

The infection of rabbits (gr B) induced an elevation in IgG1 level (0.63±0.02) relative to normal rabbits gr (0.22±0.03). In comparison to the normal rabbits (gr A), immunization with Antigen (gr C) had an extreme significant effect on IgG1 *(P<0.01)* increasing its level to be 0.76±0.12. When the immunized rabbits with Antigen were infected with 25 metacercariae (gr D), the serum IgG1 recorded 0.85±0.15, showing a highly significant elevation *(P<0.01)* than the infected control (gr B) (0.63±0.02).

Data indicated that only infection caused a significant elevation in the IgG2 level (0.66±0.12) in comparison to normal control gr (0.31±0.11). The IgG2 level in sera of rabbits immunized with Antigen (gr C) (0.91±0.13) showed a very highly significant elevation *(P<0.001)* relative to normal rabbits (gr A). Serum IgG2 level of gr D recorded 1.03±0.02, that considered a significant increase *(P<0.05)* than the level of the infected control gr (gr B) (0.66±0.12).

Although the level of IgG4 in infected control gr recorded a highly significant elevation *(P<.0.05)* (0.77±0.06), immunization of rabbits with Antigen alone (gr C) recorded a very highly significant increase *(P<0.001)* (0.97±0.021) in comparison to uninfected control gr (0.30±0.02). In case of gr D, in which rabbits were preimmunized with Antigen, then infected with *F. gigantica* metacercariae, the IgG4 levels recorded a highly significant *(P<0.01)* jump recording the highest level between all grs (1.32±0.11) in comparison to the normal or infected control gr.

F. gigantica infection induced an elevation in IL-6 level as measured in sera of infected rabbits (gr B) recording 122.21±32.30, relative to normal rabbits (gr A) which recorded 15.61±3.09. On the other hand, the IL-6 level in sera of Antigen immunized rabbits with Antigen (gr C) was 55.17±6.9. These data showed a highly significant increase *(P<0.001)* in comparison to the normal uninfected control gr. When the immunized rabbits were then infected with 25 metacercariae (gr D), the serum IL-6 level recorded 67.81±5.32, indicating slight increase in its level than the immunized gr (gr C) and recorded a significant decrease than infected gr (gr B) (122.21±32.30). Relative to normal control rabbits (gr A), data showed an increase in IL-10 level in infected control animals (gr B) (91.10±7.19 and 465.63±11.34, respectively). The IL-10 level showed a very highly significant increase *(P<0.001)* when rabbits were treated with Antigen (144.21±12.14) in comparison to control rabbits (gr A). The maximum level was obtained in rabbits immunized with Antigen and then infected (542.62±23.90) which was found to be statistically highly significant *(P<0.01)* in comparison to infected control gr.

Infection causes an increase in the level of IL-12 (110.54±10.51) (gr B) as compared to normal uninfected control gr (gr A) (30.17±1.29). The present study revealed that immunization of rabbits with purified Antigen had a significant *(P<0.05)* effect increasing IL-12 level to be

43.11±4.32. On the other hand, immunization with Antigen before infection caused a significant decrease *(P<0.01)* of the IL-12 level in serum (61.31±14.11) in comparison to infected control rabbits (gr B) (110.54±10.51).

There was an elevation in TNF-α level (541.61±25.32) as measured in rabbits infected with *F. gigantica* (gr B) in comparison to normal uninfected control gr (290.42±12.21). Treatment with purified Antigen, detected that there is a mild significant decrease in TNF-α level in immunized rabbits (288.32±50.20). Similarly, infection after Antigen prophylaxis administration recorded a significant decrease (P<0.05) in the level of serum TNF-α (321.22±12.13) as compared to infected animals (gr B) (541.61±25.32).

Discussion

Fascioliasis, an infectious parasitic disease caused by *F. hepatica* or *F. gigantica*, affects millions of people worldwide. Up to 17 million people are infected and around 91.1 million are at risk of infection **(Keiser and Utzinger, 2005)**. Today, fascioliasis is recognized as an emerging and re-emerging vector (ungulate)-borne disease with the widest latitudinal, longitudinal and altitudinal distribution known for any zoonotic disease. Hence, the World Health Organization has classified fascioliasis as an important human parasitic disease that merits international attention **(Mas-Coma et al., 2005)**. Most of the people affected by this zoonosis are in the Andean Region of South America **(Marcos et al., 2008)**. In particular, in past decades more than 1700 people in Peru have been reported to be infected by *F. hepatica* **(Marcos et al., 2007)**. Fascioliasis is an important public health problem in these regions and deserves more attention **(Marcos et al., 2009)**. Humans are often infected in communities where there is close human–ruminant interaction, such as in some South American communities, Egypt and Iran **(Jayaraj et al., 2009)**.

Triclabendazole is the only effective drug against early stages of the parasite; however, resistance to it has been extensively reported **(Villa-Mancera et al., 2008)**. Other control measures such as early diagnosis and vaccination should be developed for sustainable control of this disease that will be a cheaper, more efficient and reliable long term solution for the prevention of infection and eradication of its transmission. Diagnosis in human is based on the findings the characteristic eggs in stool and duodenal fluids **(Garacia, 2001)**. However, negative results do not rule out infection, especially in endemic areas or in field surveys undertaken for exposed agricultural community personnel **(Sabry and Mohamed, 2007)**.

The tegument of bile-dwelling *F. gigantica* is the interfacing layer that helps the parasite to maintain its homeostasis, and evade the hostile environment, including the host's immune attacks. So, some studies reported that the tegument can work as a basis for the developments of immunodiagnosis and vaccine **(Sobhon et al., 1998)**.

The present study was done to evaluate a highly sensitive and specific antigen for early diagnosis of fascioliasis and to study the humoral and cellular immune response of Antigen for developing a vaccine against this disease. These were achieved through detection of Antigen in naturally infected cattle sera using sandwich ELISA technique and vaccination of rabbits by using Antigen to prevent the infection and to eradicate its transmission.

In the present study, the purification procedure of antigen was carried out by two steps: DEAE-Sephadex G-25 and G-200 ion exchange chromatography **(Timanova et al., 1999)**. The yield was purified Antigen with protein content equal to 2.6 mg/ml, giving enough pure antigens to be used subsequently for the protection experiments. The purified Antigen appeared as a single band at 97 kDa by reducing SDS-PAGE. The results were reasonable in comparison with that was done before of purified antigen from any biological fluid following similar purification procedures **(Cancela et al., 2004)**, which purified, characterized and immunolocalized the Antigen from adult stage of *F. hepatica*.

The first step was done for preparation of pAb against *Fasciola* Antigen by immunization of rabbits with purified Antigen. The purification procedure was carried out by two steps; ammonium sulfate precipitation, and caprylic acid treatment. The prepared anti-*Fasciola* pAb was improved with protein content 10 mg/ml, mainly gamma protein. The purified pAb appeared as a double band as 31 and 53 kDa by reducing SDS-PAGE. These yields were valuable as compared with that of purified Ig following similar purification procedures which were done by **Perosa et al.** (1990), to purify the human pAb using ammonium sulfate precipitation, and caprylic acid treatment. This two-step non-chromatographic procedure was highly efficient for the purification of IgG, IgA, and IgM, thus offering several advantages over other methods of purification.

In the present work, the purified pAb against *Fasciola* Antigen was labeled with HRP conjugate (periodate method) **(Tijssen and Kurstak, 1984)**, and used as a conjugate in sandwich ELISA to immunodiagnose the fascioliasis infection in cattle. This data was confirmed with **El-Amir et al. (2008b)** who labeled pAb against *Fasciola* excretory-secretory (E/S) antigens and used it to demonstrate the presence of highly reactive epitopes on the different life cycle stages of *F. gigantica*, as well as on the different organs and PBMNCs of naturally infected cattle.

Recent studies on fascioliasis focused on the importance of ELISA in diagnosis of animal fascioliasis and it becomes the most widely used test, because of its simplicity, reliability and easy mechanization **(Awad et al., 2009)**.

Standardization of the sandwich ELISA showed that, although the optimum concentration of coating with purified pAb was only 10 µg/ml protein/well and the optimum working concentration of peroxidase conjugated anti-*Fasciola* Antigen pAb was 25µg/ml, they are enough effective indicating ideal and perfect assessment of purification techniques. To establish the sensitivity and linearity of the assay, a standard curve was plotted using *Fasciola* Antigen at concentrations 0.001-10µg/ml. The lower detection limit of the assay was 2.5µg/ml *Fasciola* Antigen which detect high efficacy of ELISA technique in this study, these data were confirmed with **El-Amir et al. (2008a)** who evaluated the diagnostic potential of different immunological techniques using *F. gigantica* E/S antigens in sheep, where the standardization of sandwich ELISA showed that, the optimum concentration of coating with purified pAb was 20 mg/dl protein/well and the optimum working concentration of peroxidase conjugated anti-E/S *Fasciola* pAb was 10 mg/dl. While, the sensitivity and linearity for the standard curve of the assay, using *Fasciola* E/S antigens at concentration 0.01-30 µg/ml was set up. The lower detection limit of the assay was 0.3 µg/ml *Fasciola* E/S antigens.

In the present study, 135 cattle blood samples were collected for the experiment after detection of adult worm in the dissected liver of naturally infected cattle. They were classified according to clinical examination into three main grs: fascioliasis (75), healthy control (30), and other parasites (30). Fascioliasis gr were classified according to parasitological investigations (egg count/g) into two grades of intensity of infection; heavy (33) (64 epg), and light infection (17) (25 epg), while 25 animals gave false negative results. Other parasitic infected gr was classified into schistosomiasis gr (10), hydatid gr (10), and hookworm gr (10).

Rabia *et al.* (2010) collected the 152 stool samples from sheep after slaughtering, then Kato-Katz concentration and Formal-Ether sedimentation techniques were performed for all stool samples in order to identify *Fasciola* eggs or other helminthic ova. *Fasciola* eggs were detected in 78 sheep (80.62%) with egg load ranging from 18-80 egg/gm stool, while other parasites including schistosomiasis, echinococcosis, anclystomiasis and ascariasis were detected in 30 sheep. Also, **El-Aziz *et al.* (2001)** collected 200 blood and fecal samples from 114 Egyptian buffaloes, 68 native breed cattle and 18 imported cattle, they were examined parasitologically for *Fasciola* infection, the result revealed that 38 (33.33%) buffaloes and 18 (26.50%) native breed cattle were positive, while all imported cattle were free from *Fasciola*. Several *F. gigantica* antigens with immunodiagnostic potential have been identified in preparations of the flukes and their E/S products **(Espino and Finaly, 1994)**. The majority of antigenic proteins derived from the surface membrane and the tegument are of 97, 66, 58, 54, 47 and 14 kDa. While, those released from the caecum are 27 and 26 kDa. These antigenic proteins include antioxidant enzyme, GST, FABP, membrane protein, hemoprotein and CP, as well as, muscle protein Antigen **(Farahnak *et al.*, 2010)** that can work as a basis for the developments of immunodiagnosis and vaccine.

In fascioliasis gr included in the present study, the sensitivity of sandwich ELISA for detection of Antigen in sera was 97.33%, while the specificity was 95%, in comparison to parasitological examination which gave 66.66% sensitivity and 100% specificity. These results indicate that the sandwich ELISA is highly sensitive and specific method for immunodiagnosis of fascioliasis. The importance of such fact is that clinically it is vital to diagnose fascioliasis as early as possible to avoid all the complications of such a disease. This is in agreement with **EL Ridi *et al.* (2007)**, who reported that *F. gigantica* E/S can be used for immunodiagnosis and prevention of sheep fascioliasis. Nine bands were apparent, the most prominent of which were 62-60, 40, 30 and 28 kDa. The data indicated that E/S-based indirect ELISA reached

100% sensitivity and specificity in immunodiagnosis of sheep fascioliasis. Also, **Kumar et al. (2008)** evaluated 27 kDa glycoprotein from somatic antigen of *F. gigantica* as a potential candidate for detection of *F. gigantica* infection in buffaloes by indirect ELISA, it was found that, the sensitivity of 27 kDa was 81%, while the specificity was 97-98% in detection of both *F. gigantica* and *F. hepatica* infections.

There is a degree of cross reactivity that was revealed in the present study between *F. gigantica* Antigen and other parasites with varying degrees, mainly schistosomiasis and hydatid, where considerable cross reactivity. This is in agreement with **Hassan et al. (1995)**, who reported that cross reactive antigens were shared between *Fasciola* and many parasites, namely schistosomiasis and echinococcosis, as well as hydatidosis **(Dalimi et al., 2004)**.

In the present study, the detection of Antigen in naturally-infected cattle sera by sandwich ELISA showed that the highest mean O.D readings were increased by the degree of infection from light to heavy infection. In other parasite grs, the highest readings were observed with *Hydatid* 2 cases out of 10, followed by *Schistosoma* 1 case out of 10, while there is no cross-reactivity with *Hookworms*. Data of the present study revealed that, sandwich ELISA is a suitable technique for diagnosis of fascioliasis infections avoiding cross reactivity with other parasites by detection of circulating Antigen in the sera.

The target of this study is scheduling our protection strategy, where rabbits were divided into four grs, normal gr (not infected or immunized), infected control gr, immunized gr with Antigen (rabbits were injected with Antigen in Freund's adjuvant), Antigen immunized and infected gr. Eight wk later, all rabbit grs were sacrificed and all parasitological and immunological parameters were analyzed.

Results clearly demonstrate that the *F. gigantica* Antigen had a strong immunoprophylactic effect against *F. gigantica* in rabbits. The protective effects were evidenced as reductions in the mean worm burden and egg counts in immunized infected gr as compared to infected control gr.

Multiple immunizations of rabbits with Antigen recorded a high significant reduction in worm burden (58.4%). A reduction in worm numbers is the gold standard for anti-*F. gigantica* vaccine development as it also had an adverse effect on the liver egg count which results in lower number of eggs recovered from liver. Administration of Antigen results in a very high significant decrease in egg count (61.4%). Our findings are in agreement with that reported by **Piacenza et al. (1999)** who observed that, immunization of sheep with native CL1 or CL2 against *F. hepatica* elicited protection levels of 33% and 34% as measured by reduction of worm burdens and of 71% and 81%, reduction in egg output, respectively, while a cocktail of native CP (CL1 and CL2) induced 60% as PR reduction in fluke burden. **Gobert and**

McManus (2005) reviewed that, early vaccination studies with Antigen against *Schistosoma* infection can lead to impressive reduction of *S. japonicum* (Philippine strain) worm burdens (mean PR of 72.6%) in mice immunized with purified Antigen from adult worms. Also, **Chen et al. (2000)** reported that, cloned full length cDNA of *S. japonicum* Antigen used to generate a recombinant vaccine. Immunization with this recombinant vaccine reduced the worm burden with 50-60% after the challenging with infection in pigs. **Jiz et al. (2008)** stated that, murine immunization studies using both biochemically purified and recombinant Antigen of *S. japonica* and *S. mansoni* have consistently demonstrated significant protection from challenge infection. Studies with *S. mansoni* demonstrated a 24 to 56% reduction in worm burdens, while protection against *S. japonicum* ranged from 32 to 86%. Maximal protection 62 to 86% against *S. japonicum* was observed by using biochemically purified Antigen followed by challenge with the Philippine strain of *S. japonicum*.

In contrast, data reported by **Muro et al. (1997)**, who tested the efficacy of *F. hepatica* rFABP as vaccine in rabbits but PR in the worm burden was not significant (11–17%) and was less than that elicited by the native molecules. Similarly, a low but significant reduction (31%) in fluke burden and 36% reduction in fluke wet weight were observed in cattle vaccinated with native FABP in CFA; however, with rFABP. This reduction in fluke burden was 1% and 11% (in CFA and Quil A, respectively) **(Estuningsih et al., 1997)**. **Ramajo et al. (2001)**, found no reduction in the worm burden in rFABP and native FABP-vaccinated sheep but there was a significant reduction in worm size and fecal egg counts, suggesting an anti-fecundity effect of the vaccine. **Raina et al. (2004)** also reported that, the antigenic stimulation by the parasite FABP to the host during the course of experimental/natural infection may not be sufficient to evoke detectable antibody level in ELISA and WB, thereby suggesting that FABP as such is a weak antigen. Also, there is no significant humoral response generated against *F. gigantica* FABP in sheep, cattle and buffaloes.

E/S-derived CL proteases were found to elicit a decrease in challenge *F. hepatica* worm burden and/or maturity in sheep **(Villa-Mancera et al., 2008)**. However, immunization of sheep with CL proteinase derived peptide led to a significant decrease in challenge *F. gigantica* worm number, but failed to influence the size of the recovered worms **(Jezek et al., 2007)**. On the other hand, the protective capacity of E/S could be related to its content of GST and FABP, major candidate vaccine antigens for fascioliasis **(McManus and Dalton, 2006)**.

Additional beneficial aspects of the protection induced by the CL vaccines were observed. First, in all vaccine trials, the proportion of liver flukes that did not develop to maturity were greater in vaccinated than in nonvaccinated controls. Consequently, the damage to the host's liver during acute infection was significantly reduced. Secondly, vaccination of both sheep and cattle also elicited a highly significant reduction (50–98%) of the parasite's ability to produce eggs, and those eggs that were synthesized showed reduced 'hatch rates' **(Mulcahy et al., 1998)**. The implications of these findings are that by reducing the parasite burden of the host and, at the same time, blocking the synthesis of viable eggs by those parasites that do survive in vaccinated animals, the vaccine would have a profound effect on pasture contamination and hence disease transmission **(Dalton et al., 2003)**.

The presented data obviously marked that the total IgG level increased with infection and during immunization with Antigen in comparison to the control grs. While on the other hand, IgM level was affected by infection and all other treatments are in close range to the infected grs. Also, IgG level was much more elevated than IgM. Thus, it may be concluded that IgG plays a prominent role in combating infection whereas IgM was not as effective.

Response of Ig isotypes between animals immunized with Antigen shows a number of differences. Antigen immunization recorded highly significant enhancement of all Ig isotypes. While, in case of immunization with Antigen followed by infection, Antigen was less potent in elevating Ig isotypes than immunization only without infection.

Bossaert et al. (2000) also found that, IgG1 was significantly higher in calves with single-dose-infected of *F. hepatica* to E/S products as compared to IgG2. **Mulcahy et al. (1998)** in their cattle immunization studies against *F. hepatica* found that, an elevation of IgG2 level was associated with protection. It is conceivable therefore that, the late strong IgG2 found in this study does put cattle better placed to eliminate the liver fluke than sheep with early and weak IgG2. However, more work needs to be done to examine the contribution of IgG2 toward protection against liver fluke.

Our results suggested that, predominance of IgG2 and IgG4 than IgG1 isotypes PI. This finding correlates with a predominance of IgG2-type Igs specific for *Fasciola spp.* antigens at different times PI. This is mostly characteristic of type 1 response which agrees with the findings of other investigators. Antibody responses in rats in the acute and chronic phase (1-21 wk) of disease show a marked predominance of IgG1 over IgG2a isotypes. During the 1st wk PI, IgG1 quickly increases, whereas, IgG2a slowly increases and reaches the highest values at 5-7 wk PI **(Gironès et al., 2007)**. **Phiri et al. (2006)** suggested that, these E/S antigens may preferentially stimulate a Th2 T cell subset response. The late IgG2 response to *F. hepatica* and *F. gigantica* E/S products in cattle may indicate a delayed Th1 T cell subset stimulation. **Moreau et al. (1998)** has previously shown that, the IgG2 response to a CL vaccine correlates with reduced worm burdens in vaccinated cattle, implying a protective role for this isotype against *F. hepatica*. These observations raise the interesting prospect that *Fasciola* parasites produce a factor (s) that can suppress IgG2 responses **(Valero et al., 2009)**.

Humans infected with *F. hepatica* develop specific antibodies of the IgM, IgA, IgE, and IgG class. **De Jesus et al. 2000** reported that, naturally occurring immunological responses to the *S. mansoni* antigens Antigen, IrV-5, Sm-23 (MAP-3), and triose phosphate isomerase (MAP-4), were evaluated. Specific IgG1, IgG2, IgG3, IgG4, and IgA levels for each of the antigens and the cytokine profile, Direct correlations between infection levels (number of epg of stool) and levels of specific IgG1 and IgG4 to SWA and Antigen were observed suggesting that these isotypes are markers for high levels of infection, while people with lower infection levels produced higher levels of IgG2 specific for these antigens. The data suggested that perhaps a vaccine that induces both Th1- and Th2-like responses would be necessary to achieve higher levels of protection.

Nara et al. (2007) suggested that, IgM, IgG2 and IgG4 initiated killing for schistosomiasis adult worms by ADCC that means it provokes an effector immune mechanism.

Our results are in agreement with that of **Zhou et al. (2000)**, who showed that pCMVSjc97 elicited much more IgG2a and IgG2b than IgG1 antibodies, whereas in mice immunized with recombinant Sjp97 protein, IgG1 was the dominant IgG subclass. Moreover, examination of cytokine production patterns revealed high level IFN-γ and IL-2 production profiles by antigen-stimulated splenocytes from pCMV-Sjc97 inoculated C57BL/6 mice. It is widely agreed that the IgG subclasses of IgG2a and IgG2b and cytokine pattern of IFN-γ and IL-2 are indicative of Th1 type responses. Thus, the profile of the immune responses induced in C57BL/6 mice by the Sjc97 nucleic acid vaccine is of a Th1-like type. It has been proved that, a Th1 type immune response generated by Sm97 is critical in the mechanism of the protection against schistosomiasis. Also, **Vazquez-Talavera et al. (2001b)** use *T. solium* Antigen as a vaccine candidate to give protection against cysticercosis in murine model; it was found that the predominant antibody isotype was IgG1 subclass that reveals production of IFN-γ and IL-2, suggesting a Th1 like profile.

In contrast, **Zhao et al. (2007)**, study the immunological response of Antigen in *Paragonimus westermani* (Pw), where the predominant antibody isotypes against recombinant PwAntigen (rPwAntigen) was IgG1 and IgG4 subclasses, suggesting that during chronic helminths infections, Th2 immune response is evoked. Also, **Garcia et al. (2008)** identified the Sm14 and Antigen epitopes that are recognized by T cells of resistant individuals living in endemic areas for schistosomiasis, it was found that protection was associated with a Th1 type of immune response induced by Sm14 peptide immunization, while immune response induced by Antigen peptide was associated with Th2 type immune response.

The Ig responses of liver fluke-infected humans to E/S antigens and to a fluke CP, CL1, showed that the predominant isotypes elicited by infection were IgG1 and IgG4, suggesting that

Th2 immune response **(O'Neill *et al.*, 1998)**. Analysis of the CL proteases-specific IgG1 antibody responses in infected cattle revealed that these antibodies do not appear in the serum until 4 or 5 wk PI. Moreover, animals given a second infection 4 wk after the primary infection did not exhibit any boosting of immune responses to the CL proteases. It is clear, therefore, that CLs are not highly immunogenic in the early stages of infection such that, at this stage, they may be considered 'hidden antigens'. This may be an important strategy used by the parasite to prevent antibodies being generated to critical molecules **(Mulcahy *et al.*, 1998)**. While the extramuscular isoforms of Antigen exist in larval stages of *S. japonica* **(Cancela *et al.*, 2004)**, thus work with both animal models and humans has strongly supported Antigen as a lead vaccine candidate for *S. mansoni and S. japonicum* **(Jiz *et al.*, 2008)**.

On the other hand, results of this thesis clearly demonstrate that immunization with Antigen elevate secretion of type 1 cytokines (IL-6, IL-12 and TNF-α) and type 2 cytokines (IL-10 levels) than the normal control gr. Administration of Antigen induces a high significant increase in IL-6 and IL-10, while, a significant increase in IL-12 and TNF-α level in immunized grs with IL-10 predominating. In contrast, there is suppression in all cytokines level in rabbits immunized with Antigen and infected grs except IL-10, which was elevated than the infected control gr. Thus, it could be hypothised that, Antigen was potent in increasing the levels of all cytokines understudy except IL-6 before infection. While, infection post immunization with Antigen caused a decrease in all cytokines except for IL-10 which remained slightly but significantly elevated.

The data presented in this study are supported by the idea of **Elizabeth and Molina (2005)** who observed that, cattle and buffaloes infected with *F. gigantica* had a predominant Th2 response which started early in the infection. IL-6 production in these animals apparently influenced the initiation and maintenance of type 2 immune response, thereby down-regulating Th1 response. IL-6 and IL-8 (in buffaloes) during infection with *F. gigantica* may thus be capable of exerting a cytotoxic effect against the fluke.

IL-6 and IL-8 have been shown to be involved in ADCC involving neutrophils. In fascioliasis, ADCC has been considered to be a mechanism by which flukes are destroyed, with the priming of neutrophils, macrophages, Eo and mast cells by various cytokines **(Hansen *et al.*, 1999; Piedrafita *et al.*, 2007)**. Therefore, cattle, buffalo and sheep, by producing IL-4, IL-6 and IL-8 during infection with *F. gigantica*, may be capable of exerting a cytotoxic effect against flukes.

In some of the infected rats, TNF-α also increased at 10 wk PI, which does not correspond to a typical Th2 response. TNF-α is implicated in the regulation of Th2 responses in other helminths infections, apparently regulating worm expulsion. Moreover, IL-4 and IL-10 can act synergistically, inhibiting the production of reactive nitrogen oxides, which up-regulate IL-12 production and inflammatory responses **(Gironès et al., 2007)**.

More recently, however, we have proposed that the secreted CLs may be involved in suppression and/or modulation of Th1 immune responses and induction of non-protective host Th2 responses **(Dixit et al., 2008)**. An analysis of cytokine production by antigen-stimulated spleen cells of *F. hepatica* infected mice showed that these are predominantly of the Th2 type, i.e. production of IL-4, IL-5 and IL-10 but little or no IFN-γ **(O'Neill et al., 2000)**. This is consistent with immunological observations in cattle which show that in the early stages of infections, mixed Th1/Th2 responses are observed but as infection progresses, a Th2 response predominates **(Mulcahy et al., 1999)**.

In conclusion, these studies proved that native heterologous *F. gigantica* Antigen significantly provides early diagnose of fascioliasis in naturally infected cattle and protects rabbits against challenge infection with *F. gigantica*. Early diagnosis using sandwich ELISA is highly sensitive and specific screening immunodiagnostic technique than parasitological examination, while multiple immunizations with native *F. gigantica* Antigen in Freund's adjuvant resulted in high significant reduction in mean worm burden and liver egg count and elicit a high significant increase in IgM and IgG antibodies, and more specifically IgG1, IgG2 and IgG4 isotypes with IgG4 isotype predominating. These data suggest that the immunoprophylactic effect of the native *F. gigantica* Antigen is mediated by a mixed Th1/Th2 response, which indicated enhancement of immune response against fascioliasis infection.

References

• **Abdel Kader A, Mostafa BB and Tantawy A. 2005.** A Field study on water characteristics and their effect on the vector snails of schistosomiasis and fascioliasis in Egypt. *J. Egypt. Ger. Soc. Zool., 48: 203-216.*

• **Abdel-Rahman S. 1996.** Immunodiagnosis of fascioliasis by detection of coproantigens. PhD Dissestation, ***Louisuna State University, Baton Rouge.***

• **Abdel-Rahman S, O'Reilly KL and Malone JB. 1999.** Biochemical characterization and localization of *Fasciola hepatica* 26-28 kDa diagnostic coproantigens. ***Parasite Immunol., 21: 279-286.***

• **Agarwal VK. 2003.** *Fasciola hepatica*: liver fluke, phylum platyhelminthes. In: Invertebrate Zoology. Agarwal VK (Ed.). Published by S. Chand and Company Ltd, Ram Nagar, ***New Delhi pp. 280-298.***

• **Allam AF, Osman MM, El-Sayed MH and Demian SR 2000.** IL1, IL-4 production and IGE levels in acute and chronic fascioliasis before and after triclabendazole treatment. *J. Egypt. Soc. Parasitol., 3: 781-790.*

• **Andrews SJ. 1999.** The life cycle of *Fasciola hepatica*. In: Fasciolosis. Dalton JP (Ed.). CAB International publishing, ***Wallingford, Oxon, UK pp. 1-21.***

• **Anuracpreeda P, Wanichanon C and Sobhon P. 2009.** *Fasciola gigantica*: Immunolocalization of 28.5 kDa antigen in the tegument of metacercaria and juvenile fluke. ***Exp. Parasitol., 122: 75-83.***

• **Arafa MS, Abaza SM, El-Shewy KA, Mohareb EW and El-Moamly AA. 1999.** Detection of *Fasciola*-specific excretory/secretory (E/S) protein fraction band (49.5 kDa) and its utilization in diagnosis of early fascioliasis using different diagnostic techniques. *J. Egypt Soc. Parasitol., 29: 11-26.*

• **Armour J and Dargie J. 1974.** Immunity to *Fasciola hepatica* in the rat. Successful transfer of immunity by lymphoid cells and serum. ***Exp. Parasitol., 35: 381–388.***

• **Armour J, Urqhart GM and Ductan JL. 1997.** Veterinary Parasitology, 2nd ed. ***Oxford: Blackwell Science Ltd, 64.***

• **Arora D and Arora B. 2005.** Trematodes a flukes in: Medical parasitolgy, 2nd ed., Satich Kumar Jain for CBS Publishers & Distributors, ***New Dehli. Banalore pp. 147.***

• **Asanji M. 1988.** The snail intermediate host of *Fasciola gigantica* and the behaviour of miracidia in host selection. ***Bull. Anim. Heal. Prod. Afr., 36: 245-250.***

- **Attallah A, Karawia E, Ismail H, Tabll A, Nawar A, Ragab A, Abdel-Aziz M and El-Dosoky I. 2002.** Identification and characterization of 26-28 kDa circulating antigen of *Fasciola gigantica*. *Ann. Trop. Med. Parasitol., 96: 271-282.*

- **Awad WS, Ibrahim AK and Salib FA. 2009.** Using indirect ELISA to assess different antigens for serodiagnosis of *Fasciola gigantica* infection in cattle, Sheep and donkeys. *Res. Vet. Sci., 86: 466-471.*

- **Barduagni P, Hassanein Y, Mohamed M, Wakeel AE, Sayed ME, Hallaj Z and Curtale F. 2008.** Use of triclabendazole for treatment of patients co-infected by *Fasciola* spp. and *S. mansoni* in Behera Governorate, Egypt. *Parasitol. Res., 102: 631-633.*

- **Barreto ML, Smith DM and Sleigh AC. 1990.** Implication of fecal egg count variation when using the Kato-Katz method to assess *Schistosoma mansoni* infection. *Trans. R. Soc. Trop. Med. Hyg., 84: 554-555.*

- **Behm CA and Sangster NC. 1999.** Pathology, Pathophysiology and Clinical Aspects. *In Dalton, J.P. (ed) Fasciolosis. CABI Publishing, Oxon, UK.*

- **Bennett CE, Hughes DL, Harness E. 1980.** *F. hepatica*: changes in tegument during killing of adult flukes surgically transferred to sensitized rats. *Parasite Immunol., 2: 93-98.*

- **Bennett CE and Threadgold LT. 1975.** *Fasciola hepatica*: Development of tegument during migration in mouse. *Exp. Parasitol., 38: 38-55.*

- **Beresain P, Goni F, Mc Gonigle S, Dowd A, Dalton J, Frangione B and Carmona C. 1997.** Proteinases secreted by *Fasciola hepatica* degrade extra-cellualr matrix and basement membrane components. *J. Parasitology, 83: 1-5.*

- **Bhamarapravati N, Thamamvill W and Limsuwan A. 1983.** Liver fluke disease of man. In: Textbook of Medicine. Edited by D.J. Weatherall, J.G.G. Ledingham, and D.D.A. Warrel, *Oxford, London.*

- **Bjorkman N and Thorsell W. 1963.** On the fine morphology of the eggshell globules in the vitelline glands of the liver fluke (*Fasciola hepatica*). *Exp. Cell Res., 32: 153-156.*

- **Boray J. 1969.** Experimental fascioliasis in Australia. *Adv. Parasitol., 7: 95-210.*

- **Boray J. 1999.** Liver fluke disease in sheep and cattle. *AgFacts, A0.9.57 (second edition), NSW Agriculture, pp15.*

- **Bossaert K, Farnir F, Leclipteux T, Protz M, Lonneux JF and Losson B. 2000.** Humoral immune-response in calves to single-dose, trickle and challenge infections with *Fasciola hepatica, Vet. Parasitol., 87: 103–123.*

- **Boyce WM, Courtney CH and Loggins PE. 1987.** Resistance to experimental infection with *F. hepatica* in exotic and domestic breeds of sheep. *Int. J. Parasitol., 17: 1233-1237.*

- **Bradford MM. 1976.** A rapid and sensitive method for the quantitation of microgram quantities of protein utilizing the principle of protein-dye binding. *Anal. Biochem., 72: 248-254.*

- **Brown WC, McElwain TF, Palmer GH, Chantler SE and Estes DM. 1999.** Bovine CD4+ T-Lymphocyte Clones Specific for Rhoptry-Associated Protein 1 of Babesia bigemina Stimulate Enhanced Immunoglobulin G1 (IgG1) and IgG2 Synthesis. *Infect. Immun. 67: 155-164.*

- **Brown WC, Woods VM, Chitko-Mckown CG, Hash SM and Rich-Ficht AC. 1994.** Interleukin-10 is expressed by bovine Type 1 helper, Type 2 helper, and unrestricted parasite-specific T-cell clones and inhibits proliferation of all three subsets in an accessory-cell-dependent manner. *Infect. Immun., 62: 4697-4708.*

- **Burden DJ, Bland AP, Hammet NC and Hughes DL. 1983.** *Fasciola hepatica*: migration of newly excysted juveniles in resistant rats. *Exp. Parasitol., 56: 277-288.*

- **Butterworth AE. 1977.** The eosinophil and its role in immunity to helminth infection. *Curr. Trop. Microbiol. Immunol., 77: 127-168.*

- **Campbell RC. 1989.** Statistics for Biologists. *3rd edition, Cambridge Univ. Press, Cambridge, New York, Melbourne, Sydney.*

- **Cancela M, Carmona C, Rossi S, Frangione B, Goñi F and Berasain P. 2004.** Purification, characterization, and immunolocalization of proteases from the adult stage of *Fasciola hepatica*. *Parasitol Res., 92: 441-448.*

- **Carmona C, Dowd A, Smith A and Dalton J. 1993.** Cathepsin-L proteinases selected by *Fasciola hepatica in vitro* prevent antibody-mediated eosinophils attachment to newly excysted juveniles. *Mol. Biochem. Parasitol., 62: 9-18.*

- **Castro E, Freyre A and Hernandez Z. 2000.** Serological responses of cattle after treatment and during natural re-infection with *Fasciola hepatica*, as measured with dot-ELISA system. *Vet. Parasitol., 90: 201-208.*

- **Cervi L, Rossi G and Masih DT. 1999.** Potential role for excretory-secretory forms of glutathione-S-transferase (GST) in *Fasciola hepatica*. *Parasitol., 119: 627-633.*

- **Chapman CB and Mitchell GF. 1982a.** Proteolytic cleavage of immunoglobulin by enzymes released by *Fasciola hepatica*. *Vet. Parasitol., 11: 165-178.*

- **Chapman CB and Mitchell GF. 1982b.** *Fasciola hepatica*: Comparative studies on fascioliasis in rat and mice. *Int. J. Parasitol., 12: 81-91.*
- **Chauvin A and Boulard C. 1996.** Local immune response to experimental *Fasciola hepatica* infection in Sheep. *Parasite, 3: 209-215.*
- **Chauvin A, Bouvet G and Boulard C. 1995.** Humoral and cellular immune responses to *Fasciola hepatica* experimental primary and secondary infection in sheep. *Int. J. Parasitol., 25: 1227–1241.*
- **Chen H, Nara T, Zeng X, Satoh M, Wu G, Jiang W, Yi F, Kojima S, Zhang S and Hirayama K. 2000.** Vaccination of domestic pig with recombinant proteases against *Schistosoma japonicum* in China. *Vaccine, 18: 2142-2146.*
- **Chensue SW, Bienkowski M, Essalu TE, Warmington KS, Hershey SP, Lukacs NW and Kunkel SI. 1993.** Endogenous IL-1 receptor antagonist regulates *Schistosoma* egg granuloma formation and regional lymphoid responses. *J. Immunol., 151: 3654-3661*
- **Cho SY, Yang HN, Kong Y, Kim JC, Shin KW and Koo BS. 1994.** Intraocular fascioliasis: a case report. *Am. J. Trop. Med. Hyg., 50: 349–353.*
- **Clery D and Mulcahy G. 1998.** Lymphocyte and cytokine responses of young cattle during primary infection with *Fasciola hepatica*. *Res. Vet. Sci., 65: 169–171.*
- **Clery D, Torgerson P and Mulcahy G. 1996.** Immune responses of chronically infected adult cattle to *Fasciola hepatica*. *Internat. J. Parasitol., 62: 71-82.*
- **Córdova M, Reátegui L and Espinoza J. 1999.** Immunodiagnosis of human fascioliasis with *Fasciola hepatica* cysteine proteinases. *Trans. R. Soc. Trop. Med. Hyg., 93: 54-57.*
- **Cox FEG, Wakelin D, Stephen HG and Dickson DD. 2005.** Melissa R, Haswell E, Lung and liver flukes In: Topley & Wilson's, microbiology and microbial infections; 10th edition, ***Hobber Arnold, London, pp: 652.***
- **Cruz-Mendoza I, Naranjo-García E, Quintero-Martínez MT, Ibarra-Velarde F and Correa D. 2006.** Exposure to *Fasciola hepatica* miracidia increases the sensitivity of *Lymnaea (Fossaria) humilis* to high and low pH. *J. Parasitol., 92: 650-652.*
- **Cuperlovic K and Movsesijan M. 1972.** Isolation and labeling of *Fasciola hepatica* antigen active during the infection. *J. Parasitol., 58: 1209-1210.*
- **Da-Costa C, Dreyfuss G, Rakotondravavao C, Rondelaud D and Da costa C. 1994.** Several observations concerning cercarial shedding of *Fasciola gigantica* from *Lymnaea natalensis*. *Parasite, 1: 39-44.*

- **Dalimi AH, Hadighi R and Madani R. 2004.** Partially purified fraction (PPF) antigen from adult *Fasciola gigantica* for the serodiagnosis of human fascioliasis using Dot-ELISA technique. *Ann. Saudi Med., 24: 18-20.*

- **Dalton JP, McGonigle S, Rolph TP and Andrews SJ. 1996.** Induction of protective immunity in cattle against infection with *Fasciola hepatica* by vaccination with cathepthin L proteinases and hemoglobin. *Infect. Immunit., 64: 5066-5074.*

- **Dalton JP, O. Neill S, Stack C, Collins P, Walshe A, Sekiya M, Doyle S, Mulcahy G, Hoyle D, Brennan G, Mousley A, Kreshchenko N, Maule AG and Donnelly SM. 2003.** *Fasciola hepatica* cathepsin L-like proteases: biology, function, and potential in the development of first generation liver fluke vaccines. *Int. J. Parasitol., 33: 1173-1181.*

- **Dalton JP, Tom TD and Strand M. 1985.** *Fasciola hepatica* comparison of immature and mature immunoreactive glycoprotein. *Parasitol. Immunol., 7: 643-657.*

- **Davies C and Goose J. 1981.** Killing of newly excysted juveniles of *Fasciola hepatica* in sensitized rats. *Parasite Immunol., 3: 81-69.*

- **De Jesus AR, Arau´ Jo I, Bacellar OV, Magalha˜ Es A, Pearce E, Harn D, Strand M and Carvalho EM. 2000.** Human Immune Responses to *Schistosoma mansoni* Vaccine Candidate Antigens. *Infect. Immun., 68: 2797–2803.*

- **De-Vias SI, Gryseels B, Van Oortmerssen GJ, Poldrman AM and Habbema JD. 1992.** A model for variations in single and repeated egg counts in *Schistosoma mansoni* infections. *J. Parasitol., 104: 451-460.*

- **Deelder AM and Ploem JS. 1975.** An immunofluorescence reaction for *Fasciola hepatica* using the defined antigen subtracts sheres system. *Exp. Parasitol., 37: 173-178.*

- **Dixit AK, Dixit P and Sharma R. 2008.** Immunodiagnostic/protective role of cathepsin L cysteine proteinases secreted by Fasciola species. *Vet. Parasitol., 154: 177-184.*

- **Dixon KE. 1966.** The physiology of excystment of the metacercariae of *Fasciola hepatica*. *Parasitol., 56: 431-456.*

- **Dowd AJ, Smith AM, McGonigle S and Dalton JP. 1994.** Purification and characterization of a second cathepsin L proteinase secreted by the parasitic trematode *Fasciola hepatica*. *Eur. J. Biochem. 233: 91-98.*

- **Doy TG and Hughes DL. 1980.** Evidence for two distinct mechanisms of resistance in the rat to reinfection with *Fasciola hepatica*. *Int. J. Parasitol., 12: 357-361.*

- **Doy TG, Hughes DL and Harness E. 1978.** Resistance of the rat to reinfection with *Fasciola hepatica* and the possible involvement of intestinal eosinophil leucocytes. *Res. Vet. Sci., 25: 41-44.*
- **Doy TG, Hughes DL, Harness G. 1981.** Hypersensitivity in rat infected with *F. hepatica:* possible role of protection against challenge infection. *Res. Vet. Sci., 30: 360-363.*
- **Dreyfuss G and Rondelaud D. 1997.** *Fasciola gigantica* and *Fasciola hepatica*: A comparative study of some characteristics of *Fasciola* infection in *Lymnaea truncatula* infected by either of the two trematodes. *Vet. Res., 28: 123–130.*
- **Duffus WPH and Frankes D. 1980.** In vitro effect of immune serum and bovine granulocytes on juvenile *Fasciola hepatica. Clin. Exp. Immunol., 41: 430-437.*
- **Duménigo BE, Espino AM and Finlay CM. 1996.** Detection of *F. hepatica* antigen in cattle faeces by a monoclonal-based sandwich immunoassay. *Res. Vet. Sci., 60: 278-279.*
- **Dunne DW. 1990.** Schistosome carbohydrate. *Parasitol. Today, 6: 45-48.*
- **El-Amir A, Rabee I, Kamal N and El-Deeb S. 2008a.** Evaluation of the diagnostic potential of different immunological techniques using polyclonal antibodies against *Fasciola gigantica* excretory/secretory antigens in sheep. *Egypt. J. Immunol., 15: 65-74.*
- **El-Amir A, Rabee I, Mohamed D and El-Deeb S. 2008b.** Immunolocalization of excretory/secretory antigens expressed on different life cycle stages of *Fasciola gigantica* and in different organs of infected cattle. *Proc. Zool. Soc. A.R. Egypt., 50: 135-158.*
- **El-Aziz MM, Ghazy AA, Effat MM. 2001.** Immunodiagnosis of bovine fasciolosis using *F. hepatica* excretory-secretory antigens ELISA. *J. Egypt Soc. Parasitol., 31: 327-334.*
- **El-Bahy MM, Malone JB and Todd WL. 1992.** Detection of stable diagnostic antigen in the bile and feces of *Fasciola hepatica* infected cattle. *Vet. Parasitol., 45: 157-167.*
- **EL-Kerdany ED, Abd-Alla NM and Sharaki OA. 2002.** Recognition of antigenic components of *Fasciola gigantica* their use in immunodiagnosis. *J. Egypt. Soc. Parasitol., 32: 675-690.*
- **Elizabeth C and Molina J. 2005.** Serum interferon-gamma and interleukins-6 and -8 during infection with *Fasciola gigantica* in cattle and buffaloes. *Vet. Sci., 6: 135–139.*
- **El Ridi R, Salah M, Wagih A, William H, Tallima H, El Shafie MH, Abdel Khalek T, El Amir A, Abo Ammou FF, and Motawi H. 2007.** *Fasciola gigantica*

excretory/secretory products for immunodiagnosis and prevention of sheep fasciolosis. *Vet. Parasitol.*, *149: 219-228.*

• **Engels D, Nathimana S, De-Vias SJ and Gryseels B. 1997.** Variation in weight of stool samples prepared by the Kato-Katz method and its implications. *Trop. Med. Internat. Health, 2: 265-271.*

• **Engvall E and Perlmanm P. 1971.** Enzyme-linked immunosorbent assay. Quantitative assay of IgG. *Immunochem., 8: 871-874.*

• **Ericksen L and Flagsted T. 1974.** *Fasciola hepatica*: Influence of extrahepatic adult flukes on infections and immunity in rats. *Exp. Parasitol., 35: 411-417.*

• **Espino AM and Finlay CM. 1994.** Sandwich enzyme-linked immunosorbent assay for deection of excretory-secretory antigens in humans fascioliasis by sandwich enzyme-linked immunosorbent assay. *J. Clin. Microbiol., 32: 190-193.*

• **Espino AM, Marcet R and Finlay CM. 1990.** Detection of circulating excretory antigens in human fascioliasis by sandwich enzyme-linked immunosorbent assay. *J. Clin. Microbiol., 28: 2637-2640.*

• **Espino AM, Marcet R and Finlay CM. 1997.** *F. hepatica*: Detection of antigenemia and coproantigens in experimentally infected rats. *Exper. Parasitol., 85: 117–120.*

• **Esteban JG, Gonzalez C and Curtale F. 2003.** Hyperendemic fascioliasis associated with schistosomiasis in villages in the Nile Delta of Egypt. *Am. J. Trop. Med. Hyg., 69: 429-434.*

• **Estuningsih SE, Smooker PM, Wiedosari E, Widjajant S, Viano S, Partoutomo S and Spithill TW. 1997.** Evaluation of antigens of *Fasciola giogantica* as vaccines against tropical fascioliasis in cattle. *Internat. J. Parasitol., 27: 1419-1428.*

• **Fagbemi BO, Aderibigbe OA and Guobadia EE. 1997.** The use of monoclonal antibody for the immunodiagnosis of *Fasciola gigantica* infection in cattle. *Vet. Parasitol., 69: 231-240.*

• **Fagbemi BO and Guobadia EE. 1995.** Immunodiagnosis of fascioliasis in ruminants using a 28-kDa cysteine protease of *F. gigantica* adult worm. *Vet. Parasitol., 57: 309-318.*

• **Fagbemi BO and Hillyer GV. 1991.** Partial purification and characterization of the Proteolytic enzymes of *Fasciola gigantica* adult worms. *Vet. Parasitol., 40: 217-226.*

• **Fagbemi BO and Hillyer GV. 1992.** The purification and characterization of a cysteine protease of adult worms. *Vet. Parasitol., 43: 223-232.*

- **Fagbemi BO, Obarisiagbon IO and Mbuh JV. 1995.** Detection of circulating antigen in sera of *Fasciola gigantica* infected cattle with antibodies reactive with a *Fasciola*-specific 88-Kda antigen. *Vet. Parasitol., 58: 235-246.*

- **FAO. 1997.** *Home page at http://apps.fao.org/lim soo l nph_wrap.pl.*

- **Farahnak A, Golmohamadi T and Molaei Rad MB. 2010.** Carbohydrate detection and lectin isolation from tegumental tissue of *Fasciola hepática*. *Iranian J Parasitol., 5: 20-24.*

- **Flynn RJ, Mannion C, Golden O, Hacariz O and Mulcahy G. 2007.** Experimental *Fasciola hepatica* infection alters responses to tests used for diagnosis of bovine tuberculosis. *Infect. Immun., 75: 1373-1381.*

- **Fonseca CT, Brito CF, Alves JB and Oliveira SC. 2004.** IL-12 enhances protective immunity in mice engendered by immunization with recombinant 14 kDa *Schistosoma mansoni* fatty acid-binding protein through an IFN-γ and TNF-α dependent pathway. *Vaccine, 22: 503-510.*

- **Gajewska A, Smaga-Kozlowska K and Wisniewski M. 2005.** Pathological changes of liver in infection of *Fasciola hepatica*. *Wiad Parazytol., 51: 115-23.*

- **Ganga G, Varshney JP, Sharma RL and Kalicharan A. 2007.** Effect of Fasciola infection on adrenal and thyroid glands of riverine buffaloes. *Res. Vet. Sci., 82: 61-67.*

- **Garcia LS. 2001.** Liver and lung trematodes. In: Diagnostic Medical Parasitology. *Garcia LS (Ed.). 4th edition. American Society for Microbiology Press, NW, Washington, DC, USA pp. 433-436.*

- **Garcia TC, Fonseca CT, Pacifico LG, Durães Fdo V, Marinho FA, Penido ML, Caliari MV, de Melo AL, Pinto HA, Barsante MM, Cunha-Neto E and Oliveira SC. 2008.** Peptides containing T cell epitopes, derived from Sm 14, but not from proteases, induce a Th1 type of immune response, reduction in liver pathology and partial protection against *Schistosoma mansoni* infection in mice. *Acta Trop., 106: 162-167.*

- **Garraud O and Nutman TB. 1996.** The role of cytokines in human B-cell differentiation into immunoglobulin-secreting cells. *Bul. Inst. Pasteur., 94: 285-309.*

- **Garraud O, Perraut R, Riveau G and Nutman TB. 2003.** Class and subclass selection in parasite-specific antibody responses. *Trends Parasitol., 19: 300-304.*

- **Ghosh S, Rawat P, Velusamy R, Joseph P, Gupta SC and Singh BP. 2005.** 27kDa *Fasciola gigantica* glycoprotein for the diagnosis of prepatent fasciolosis in cattle. *Vet. Res. Commun., 29:123-135.*

- Gironès N, Valero MA, García-Bodelón MA, Chico-Calero I, Punzón C, Fresno M and Mas-Coma S. 2007. Immune suppression in advanced chronic fascioliasis: an experimental study in a rat model. *J. Infect. Dis.*, *195: 1504-1512.*

- Gobert GN and McManus DP. 2005. Update on proteases in parasitic worms. *Parasitol. Internat., 54: 101-107.*

- Goose J. 1978. Possible role of excretory/secretory production in evasion of host defenses by *Fasciola hepatica*. *Nature, 275: 216-217.*

- Guobadia EE and Fagbemi BO. 1995. Time-course analysis of antibody response by EITB and ELISA before and after chemotherapy in sheep infected with *Fasciola gigantica*. *Vet. Parasitol., 58: 247-253.*

- Guobadia EE and Fagbemi BO. 1996. Detection of circulating *F. gigantica* antigen in experimental and natural infections of sheep with fasciolosis. *Vet. Parasitol., 65: 29-39.*

- Guralp N, Ozcan C and Simms BT. 1964. *Fasciola gigantica* and fascioliasis in Turkey. *Am. J. Vet. Res., 25: 196-210.*

- Hammouda NA, el Mansoury ST, el Azzouni MZ and Hussein ED. 1997. Detection of circulating antigens in blood to evaluate treatment of fascioliasis. *J. Egypt. Soc. Parasitol., 27: 365-371.*

- Hanna REB. 1980. *F. hepatica*: An immunofluorescent study of antigenic changes in the tegument during development in the rat and sheep. *Exp. Parasitol., 50: 155-170.*

- Hansen D, Clery D, Estuningsih S, Widjajanti S, Partoutomo S and Spithill T. 1999. Immune responses in Indonesian thin tail and Merino sheep during a primary infection with *Fasciola gigantica*: lack of a specific IgG2 antibody response is associated with increased resistance to infection in Indonesian sheep. *Int. J. Parasitol., 29: 1027–1035.*

- Haridy FM, El-Garhy M and Morsy TA. 2003. Efficacy of miarzid (Commiphora molmol) against fascioliasis in Egyptian sheep. *J. Egypt Soc. Parasitol., 33: 917-924.*

- Haridy FM, Ibrahim BB, Morsey TA and El-Sharkawy IM. 1999. Fascioliasis an increasing zoonotic disease in Egypt. *J. Egypt Soc. Parasitol., 29: 35-448.*

- Haroun EM and Hillyer GV. 1986. Resistance to fascioliasis- a review. *Vet. Parasitol., 20: 63-93.*

- Haroun EM, Hammond JA and Sewell MM. 1980. Resistance to *Fasciola hepatica* in rats and rabbits following sensitizing infection and treatment. *Res. Vet. Sci., 28: 377-379.*

- **Haseeb AN, EL-Shazly AM, Arafa MA and Morsy AT. 2002.** A review on fascioliasis in Egypt. *J. Egypt Soc. Parasitol., 32: 317-354.*
- **Haseeb AN, El-Shazly AM, Arafa MA and Morsy AT. 2003.** Evaluation of excretory/secretory *Fasciola antigen* in diagnosis of human fascioliasis. *J. Egypt. Soc. Parasitol., 33: 123-138.*
- **Hassan MM, Moustafa NE, Mahmoud LA, Abbaza BE and Hegab MH. 1995.** Prevalence of *Fasciola* infection in school children in Sharkia governate, Egypt. *J. Egy. Soc. Parasitol., 25: 543-549.*
- **Heussler VT and Dobbelaere DA. 1994.** Cloning of a protease gene family of *Fasciola hepatica* by polymerase chain reaction. *Mol. Biochem. Parasitol., 64: 11-23.*
- **Hillyer GV. 1999.** Immunodiagnosis of human and animal fasciolosis. In: Fasciolosis. *Dalton JP (Ed.). CAB International publishing, Wallingford, Oxon, UK pp 435-442.*
- **Hillyer GV and de-Ateca LS. 1979.** Immunity in *Schistosoma mansoni* using antigens of Fasciola hepatica isolated by concanavalin A affinity chromatography. *Infect. Immunity., 26: 802-807.*
- **Hillyer GV and Soler de Galanes M. 1991.** Initial feasibility studies of the FAST-ELISA for the immunodiagnosis of fascioliasis. *J Parasitol. 77: 362-365.*
- **Hillyer GV, Soler de Galanes M and Battisti G. 1992a.** *F. hepatica*: host responders and nonrespnders to parasite glutathione S-transferase. *Exp. Parasitol., 75: 176-186.*
- **Hillyer GV, Soler de Galanes M, Rodriguez-Perez J, Bjorland J, Silva de Lagrava M, Ramirez Guzman S and Bryan RT. 1992b.** Use of the Falcon assay screening test-enzyme-linked immunosorbent assay (FAST-ELISA) and the enzyme linked immunoelectrotransfere blot (EITB) to determine the prevalence of human Fascioliasis in the Bolivian Altiplano. *Am. J. Trop. Med. Hyg., 46: 603-609.*
- **Hughes DL, Harness E and Doy TG. 1981.** The different stages of *Fasciola hepatica* capable of inducing immunity and the susceptibility of various stages to immunological attack in the sensitised rat. *Res. Vet. Sci., 30: 93-98.*
- **Ibarra F, Vera Y, Quiroz H, Cantó J, Castillo R, Hernández A and Ochoa P. 2004.** Determination of the effective dose of an experimental fasciolicide in naturally and experimentally infected cattle. *Vet. Parasitol., 120: 65-74.*
- **Intapan PM, Maleewong W, Nateeworanart S, Wongkham C, Pipitgool V, Sukolapong V and Sangmaneedet S. 2003.** Immunodiagnosis of human fascioliasis

using an antigen of *Fasciola gigantica* adult worm with the molecular mass of 27 kDa by a dot-ELISA. *Southeast Asian J. Trop. Med. Public Health., 34: 713-717.*

- **Jayaraj R, Piedrafita D, Dynon K, Grams R, Spithill TW and Smooker PM. 2009.** Vaccination against fasciolosis by a multivalent vaccine of stage-specific antigens. *Vet. Parasitol., 160: 230-236.*

- **Jezek J, El Ridi R, Salah M, Wagih A, Aziz HW, Tallima H, El Shafie MH, Abdel Khalek T, Abo Ammou FF, Strongylis C, Moussis V and Tsikaris V. 2007.** *Fasciola gigantica* cathepsin L proteinase-based synthetic peptide for immunodiagnosis and prevention of sheep fasciolosis. *Biopolymers., 88: 20-28.*

- **Jiz M, Wu H-W, Meng R, Pond-Tor S, Reynolds M, Friedman JF, Olveda R, Ascota L and Kurtis JD. 2008.** Pilot-Scale Production and Characterization of Proteases, a Vaccine Candidate for *Schistosomiasis japonica*. *Infect. Immun., 76: 3164-3169.*

- **Kagan IG. 1979.** Diagnostic, Epidemiologic and Experimental Parasitology: Immunologic aspects. *Am. J. Trop. Med. Hyg., 28: 429-439.*

- **Kanoksil W, Wattanatranon D, Wilasrusmee C, Mingphruedh S and Bunyaratvej S. 2006.** Case Report Endoscopic Removal of One Live Biliary *Fasciola gigantic*a. *J. Med. Assoc. Thai., 89: 2150-2154.*

- **Keiser J and Utzinger J. 2005.** Emerging foodborne trematodiasis. *Emerging Infect. Dis., 11: 1507–1514.*

- **Kelly JD, Campbell NJ and Dineen JK. 1980.** The role of the gut in acquired resistance to *Fasciola hepatica* in the rat. *Vet. Parasitol., 6: 359-367.*

- **Kendall SB. 1974.** Some parasites of domestic animals in the Aswan Governorate-Arab Rupablic of Egypt. *Trop. Anim. Heal. Prod., 6: 128-130.*

- **Keyyu JD, Kassuku AA, Msalilwa LP, Monrad J and Kyvsgaard NC. 2006.** Cross-sectional prevalence of helminth infections in cattle on traditional, small-scale and large-scale dairy farms in Iringa district, Tanzania. *Vet. Res. Commun., 30: 45-55.*

- **Khalil HM, Abdel Aal TM, Maklad MK, Abdallah HM, Fahmy IA and EL Zayyat EA. 1990.** Specificity of crude and purified *Fasciola* antigens in immunodiagnosis of human fascioliasis. *J. Egy. Soc. Parasitol., 20: 87-94.*

- **Khalil SS, Abou Shousha S, Farahat AA and Rashwan EA. 1999.** Production of pro-inflamatory cytokines (GM-CSF, IL.8 and IL-6) by monocytes from fascioliasis patients. *J. Egypt. Soc. Parasitol., 3: 1007-1015.*

- Kim k, Yang HJ and Chung YB. 2003. Usefulness of 28 kDa protein of *Fasciola hepatica* in diagnosis of fascioliasis. ***Korean J. Parasitol., 41: 121-123.***

- Knox DP. 1994. Parasite enzyme and the control of round-worm and fluke infestation in domestic animals. ***Brit. Vet. J., 150: 319-337.***

- Kohama H, Harakuni T, Kikuchi M, Nara T, Takemura Y, Miyata T, Sato Y, Hirayama K and Arakawa T. 2010. Intranasal administration of Schistosoma japonicum proteases induced robust long-lasting systemic and local antibody as well as delayed-type hypersensitivity responses, but failed to confer protection in a mouse infection model. ***Jpn. J. Infect. Dis., 63: 166-172.***

- Kojima S. 2004. Overview: from the horse experimentation by Prof. Akira Fujinami to proteases. ***Parasitol. Internat., 53: 151-162.***

- Kumar N, Ghosh S and Gupta SC. 2008. Early detection of Fasciola gigantica in buffaloes by enzyme-linked Immunosorbent assay and dot enzyme-linked Immunosorbent assay. ***Parasitol. Res., 103: 141-150.***

- Kumar S and Sharma MC. 1991. Infertility in rural cows in relation to fascioliasis. ***Ind. J. Anim. Sci. 61: 838-840.***

- Laemmli VK. 1970. Cleavage of structural proteins during assembly of the head of the bacteriophage T4. ***Nature, 277: 630-634.***

- Langley RJ and Hillyer GV. 1989. Detection of circulating parasite antigen in murine fascioliasis by two-site enzyme-linked immunosorbent asssays. ***Am. J. Trop. Med. Hyg., 41: 472-478.***

- Laursen JR, Averbeck GA and Conboy GA. 1989. Preliminary survey of pulmonate snails of central Minnesota. ***Final report submitted to the Novagame Wildlife Program, Minnesota Department of Natural Resources. Unpaged report.***

- Leclipteuxa TH, Torgersonb PR, Dohertyb ML, McColeb D, Protza M, Farnirc F and Lossona B. 1998. Use of excretory/secretory antigens in a competition test to follow the kinetics of infection by Fasciola hepatica in cattle. ***Vet. Parasitol., 77: 103-114.***

- Levine DM, Hillyer GV and Flores SI. 1980. Comparison of counterelectrophoresis the enzyme-linked immunosorbent assay, and Kato fecal examination for the diagnosis of fascioliasis in infected mice and rabbits. ***Am. J. Trop. Med. Hyg., 29: 602-608.***

- Liu D, Lightowler M, Richard M. 1992. Evaluation of a monoclonal antibody-based competition ELISA for the diagnosis of human hydatidosis. ***Parasitol., 104: 357-361.***

- **Lopez-Moreno HS, Correa D, Laclette JP and Ortiz-Navarrette VF. 2003.** Identification of CD4+ T cell epitopes of *Taenia solium* proteases. *Parasite Immunol., 25: 513-516.*

- **Maggioli G, Piacenza L, Carambula B, and Carmona C. 2004.** Purification, characterization and immunolocalization of a thioredoxin reductase from adult *Fasciola hepatica. J. Parasitol., 90: 205–211.*

- **Maher K, El Ridi R, El-Hoda AN, El-Ghannam M, Shaheen H, Shaker Z, Hassanein HI. 1999.** Parasite-specific antibody profile in human fascioliasis: application for immunodiagnosis of infection. *Am. J. Trop. Med. Hyg., 61: 738-742.*

- **Maizels RM, Sartoro E, Kurniawan A, Partono F, Selkrik ME and Yazdanbakhsh M. 1995.** T-cell activation and the balance of antibody isotypes in human lymphatic filariasis. *Parasitol. Today, 11: 50-56.*

- **Maleewong W, Intapan PM, Wongkham C, Sripa B, Sukolapeong V and Ieamvitee vanich K. 1997.** Specific monoclonal antibodies to *Fasciola gigantica. Asian Pac. J. Alter. Immunol., 15: 49-54.*

- **Maleewong W, Intapan PM, WongKhan C, Tomanakan K, Daenseekaew W and Sukeepaisarnjaroen W. 1996.** Comparison of adult somatic and excretory–secretory antigen in enzyme–linked immunosorbent assay for serodiagnosis of human infection with *Fasciola gigantica. Southeast Asian. J. Med. Pub. Heal., 27: 566-569.*

- **Manson-Bahr PEC and Apted FIC. 1985.** In: Manson's Tropical Diseases, 18th edition. *Bailliere Tindall From and London.*

- **Mansour NS, Youssef FG, Michail EM and Boctor FN. 1983.** Use of partially purified *Fasciola gigantica* worm antigen in the serological diagnosis of human fascioliasis in Egypt. *Am. J. Trop. Med. Hyg., 32: 550-554.*

- **Marcos LA, Bussalleu A, Terashima A and Espinoza J. 2009.** Detection of antibodies against *Fasciola hepatica* in cirrhotic patients from Peru. *J. Helminthol., 83: 23-26.*

- **Marcos LA, Terashima A and Gotuzzo E. 2008.** Update on hepatobiliary flukes: fascioliasis, opisthorchiasis and clonorchiasis. *Curr. Opin. Infect. Dis., 21: 523-530.*

- **Marcos LA, Terashima A, Leguia G, Canales M and Gotuzzo E. 2007.** *F. hepatica* infection in Peru: an emergent disease. *Rev. Gastroenterol. del Peru., 27: 389-396.*

- **Marsden PD and Warren KS. 1984.** Fascioliasis. In: Warren KS, Mahmoud AAF, eds. Tropical and Geographical Medicine. *New York: McGraw-Hill; 458-460.*

- **Martinez-Moreno A, Martinez-Moreno FJ, Acosta I, Gulierrez PN, Becerra C and Hernandez S. 1997.** Humoral and cellular immune responses to experimental *Fasciola hepatica* infections in goats. *Parasitol. Res., 83: 680-686.*

- **Mas-Coma S. 2004.** Human fascioliasis (In: Waterborne Diseases: Identification, Causes and Control. (ED. Cotruvo JA, Dufour A, Rees G et al.), WHO, IWA Publishing, London, *UK, pp: 305-318.*

- **Mas-Coma S, Rodriguez A and Bargues MD. 1997.** Secondary reservoir role of domestic animals other than sheep and cattle in fascioliasis transmission in the Northern Bolivian Altiplano. *Res. Rev. Parasitol., 57: 39-46.*

- **Mas-Coma S, Bargues MD and Valero MA. 2005.** Fascioliasis and other plant-borne trematode zoonoses. *Int. J. Parasitol., 35: 1255-1278.*

- **Mas-Coma S, Esteban JG and Bargues M. 1999.** Epidemeology of human fascioliasis: A review and proposed new classification. *Bull. Wld. Hlth. Orge., 77: 340-346.*

- **Mbuh J and Fagbemi B. 1996.** Antibody and circulating antigen profiles before and after chemotherapy in goats infected with *F. gigantica*. *Vet. Parasitol., 66: 171-179.*

- **McCole DF, Doherty ML, Baird AW, Davis WC, McGill K and Torgerson PR. 1999.** T cell subset involvement in immune responses to *Fasciola hepatica* infection in cattle. *Parasite Immunol., 21: 1–8.*

- **McGonigle S and Dalton JP. 1995.** Isolation of *Fasciola hepatica* hemoglobin. *Parasitol., 111: 209-215.*

- **Mckinney MM and Parkinson A. 1987.** A simple, non-chromatographic procedure to purify immunoglobulins from ascites fluid. *J. Immunol. Meth., 96: 271-278.*

- **McManus D and Dalton J. 2006**. Vaccines against the zoonotic trematodes *Schistosoma japonicum, Fasciola hepatica* and *Fasciola gigantica*. *Parasitol., 133: 43-61.*

- **Medhat A, Shehata M, Bucci K, Mohamed S, Diab A, Dief E, Badary S, Galal H, Nafe M and Christopher LK. 1998.** Increase interleukin-4 and interleukin-5 production in response to *Schistosoma haematobium* adult worm antigens correlated with lake of reinfection after treatment. *J. Infect. Dis., 178: 512-519.*

- **Meeusen E and Brandon M. 1994.** The use of antibody-secreting cell probes to reveal tissue-restricted immune responses during infection. *Eur. J. Immunol., 24: 469–474.*

- **Meeusen ENT and Piedrafita D. 2003.** Exploiting natural immunity to helminthic parasites for the development of veterinary vaccines. *Intl. Parasitol., 33: 1285-1290.*

- **Mezo M, Gonzalez-Warleta M, Carro C and Ubeira FM. 2004.** An ultra sensitive captures ELISA for detection of *Fasciola hepatica* Coproantigens in sheep and cattle using a new monoclonal antibody (MMS). *J. Parasitol., 90: 845-852.*

- **Milbourne EA and Howell MJ. 1990.** Eosinophils response to Fasciola hepatica in rodents. *J. Parasitol., 20: 705-708.*

- **Mohsen MH, Mona AM, Nawras M, Ahmed S, Adel A and Nashwa IIR. 2002.** Dot ELISA for measuring anti-*Fasciola* IgG isotypes among patients with fascioliasis. *J. Egypt Soc. Parasitol., 32: 571-578.*

- **Molina EC and Skerratt LF. 2005.** Cellular and humoral responses in liver of cattle and buffaloes infected with a single dose of *F. gigantica*. *Vet. Parasitol., 131: 157-163.*

- **Moreau E, Chauvin A and Boulard C. 1998.** IFN-gamma and IL-10 productions by hepatic lymph node and peripheral blood lymphocytes in *Fasciola hepatica*-infected sheep. *Parasite, 5: 307-315.*

- **Morphew RM, Wright HA, Lacourse EJ, Woods DJ and Brophy PM. 2007.** Comparative proteomics of excretory-secretory proteins released by the liver fluke *Fasciola hepatica* in sheep host bile and during in vitro culture ex-host. *Mol. Cell Proteomics., 6: 963-972.*

- **Mostafa B, Abdel Kader A and Tantawy A. 2005.** Distribution of snail vectors of schistosomiasis and fascioliasis and infection risks at some rice farming sites in Kafr El-Sheikh and El-Qarbiya Governorates, Egypt: The present status. *J. Egypt. Ger. Soc. Zool., 46: 53-65.*

- **Mousa WM. 1994.** Evaluation of specific *F. gigantica* antigens for diagnosis of fascioliasis in experimentally and naturally infected sheep by ELISA. *Vet Med J 42: 77-81.*

- **Mulcahy G and Dalton JP. 1998.** Vaccines in the control of liver fluke infection in ruminants: current status and prospects. *Irish Vet. J., 51: 520-525.*

- **Mulcahy G, Joyce P and Dalton J. 1999.** Immunology of *F. hepatica* infection. In: Dalton, J.P. (Ed.), Fasciolosis. *CAB International Publishing, Wallingford, UK, 341–375.*

- **Mulcahy G, O'Connor F, McGonigle S, Dowd A, Clery D, Andrews SJ and Dalton JP. 1998.** Correlation of specific antibody titre and avidity with protection in cattle immunized against *Fasciola hepatica*. *Vaccine, 16: 932-939.*

- Muro A, Ramajo V, López J, Simón F and Hillyer GV. 1997. *Fasciola hepatica*: vaccination of rabbits with native and recombinant antigens related to fatty acid binding proteins. *Vet. Parasitol., 69: 219-229.*

- Mwatha JK, Kimani G, Kamau T, Mbugua GG, Ouma JH, Mumo J, Fulford AJ, Jones FM, Butterworth AE, Roberts MB and Dunne DW. 1998. High levels of TNF, soluble TNF receptors, soluble ICAM-1, and IFN-gamma, but low levels of IL-5, are associated with hepatosplenic disease in human schistosomiasis mansoni. *J Immunol., 160: 1992-1999.*

- Nara T, Hzumi K, Ohmae H, Sy OS, Tsubota S, Inaba Y, Tsubouchi A, Tanabe M, Kojima S and Aoki T. 2007. Antibody Isotype Responses to Proteases, A Vaccine Candidate for Schistosomiasis, and Their Correlations with Resistance and Fibrosis in Patients Infected with *Schistosoma japonicum* in Leyte, The Philippines. *Am. J. Trop. Med. Hyg., 76: 384-391.*

- Naus CW, Kimani G, Ouma JH, Fulford AJ, Webster M, Van Dam GJ, Deelder AM, Butterworth AE and Dunne DW. 1999. Development of antibody isotype responses to *Schistosoma mansoni* in an immunologically naive immigrant population: influence of infection duration, infection intensity, and host age. *Infect. Immun., 67: 3444-3451.*

- Nessim NG, Hassan SI, William S and El-Baz H. 2000. Effect of the broad spectrum anthelmintic drug flubendazole upon *Schistosoma mansoni* experimentally infected mice. *Arzneimittelforschung., 50: 1129-1133.*

- Nilsson BO. 1990. Enzyme-linked immunosorbent assay. *Curr. Opin. Immunol., 2: 898-904.*

- Nowotny A. 1979. Basic Exercises in immunochemistry. Springer Verlag, Berlin Heidelberg. *New York. pp: 7-20.*

- Oldham G and Williams L. 1985. Cell mediated immunity to liver fluke antigens during experimental *Fasciola hepatica* infection of cattle. *Parasite Immunol., 7: 503–516.*

- O'Neill SM, Brady MT, Callanan JJ, Mulcahy G, Joyce P, Mills KHG and Dalton JP. 2000. *Fasciola hepatica* infection down-regulates Th1 responses in mice. *Parasite Immunol., 22: 147-155.*

- O'Neill SM, Parkinson M, Strauss W, Angles R and Dalton JP. 1998. Immunodiagnosis of *Fasciola hepatica* infection (fascioliasis) in human population in the

Bolivian Altiplano using purified cathepsin L cysteine protease. *Am. J. Trop. Med. Hyg.,* *58: 417-423.*

- **Ortiz PL, Claxton JR, Clarkson MJ, McGarry J and Williams DJ. 2000.** The specificity of antibody response in cattle naturally exposed to *Fasciola hepatica. Vet. Parasitol., 93: 121-134.*

- **Osman MM and Abo El-Nazar SY. 1999.** Evaluation of *Fasciola* somatic antigenic fractions in the diagnosis of human fascioliasis. *J. Egy. Soc. Parasitol., 22: 27-35.*

- **Osman MM, Lausten SB, El-Sefi T, Boghdadi I, Rashed MY and Jensen SL. 1989.** Biliary Parasites. *Dig. Surg., 4: 287-296.*

- **Osman MM, Shehab AY, El-Masry SA, Helmy MH and Farag HF. 1995.** Evaluation of *Fasciola* excretory–secretory (E/S) products in diagnosis of acute human fascioliasis by IgM ELISA. *Trop. Med. Parasitol., 46: 115-118.*

- **Osman MM, Zaki A, Abutt Samra L, Farag HF and Youssef MM. 1992.** Evaluation of *Fasciola* somatic antigenic fractions in the diagnosis of human fascioliasis. *J. Egypt. Soc. Parasitol., 22: 27-35.*

- **Overend DJ and Bowen FL. 1995.** Resistance of *Fasciola hepatica* to triclabendazole. *Austral. Vet. J., 72: 275-276.*

- **Park TJ, Kang J, Na B and Sohn W. 2009.** Molecular cloning and characterization of a proteases from Clonorchis sinensis. *Korean J. Parasitol., 47: 359-367.*

- **Partoutomo S, Ronohardjo P, Wilson AJ and Stervenson P. 1985.** Review of diseases in Indonesia affecting draught power in domestic animals. In: Draught Animal Power for Production. *Copland JW (Ed.). ACIAR, Canberra, Australia pp. 140-146.*

- **Patil K, Kulkarni S, Gorad K, Panchal A, Arora S and Gautam R. 2009.** Acute Fascioliasis-Rare Cause of Obstructive Jaundice – A Case Report. *Bombay Hosp. J., 51: 398-400.*

- **Pelley RP and Hillyer GV. 1978.** Demonstration of a common antigen between *Schistosoma mansoni* and *Fasciola hepatica. Am. J. Trop. Med. Hyg., 27: 1192-1194.*

- **Perosa F, Carbone R, Ferrone S and Dammacco F. 1990.** Purification of human immunoglobulins by sequential precipitation with caprylic acid and ammonium sulphate. *J. Immunol. Methods, 128: 9-16.*

- Phiri AM, Phiri IK, Sikasunge CS, Chembensofu M and Monrad J. 2006. Comparative fluke burden and pathology in condemned and noncondemned cattle livers from selected abattoirs in Zambia. *Onderstepoort. Vet. Res., 73: 275-281.*
- Piacenza L, Acosta D, Basmadjian I, Dalton JP and Carmona C. 1999. Vaccination with cathepsin L proteinases and with leucine aminopeptidase induces high levels of protection against fascioliasis in sheep. *Infect. Immunity., 67: 1954-1961.*
- Piedrafita D, Estuningsih E, Pleasance J, Prowse R, Raadsma H, Meeusen E and Spithill T. 2007. Peritoneal lavage cells of Indonesian thin-tail sheep mediate antibody-dependent superoxide radical cytotoxicity *in vitro* against newly excysted juvenile *Fasciola gigantica* but not juvenile *Fasciola hepatica*. *Infect. Immun., 75: 1954-1963.*
- Prasitirat P, Thammasart S, Chompoochan T, Nithiuthai S and Taira S. 1996. The dynamics of antibody titres and fecal egg output in cattle and buffalo following infection with 500 and 1000 *Fasciola gigantica* metacercariae. *Thai. J. Vet. Med., 26: 85-89.*
- Pujol FH and Cesari IM. 1990. Antigenicity of adult *Schistosoma mansoni* alkaline phosphatase. *Parasite Immunol., 12: 189: 198.*
- Qureschi T, Wagner GG, Drawe DL, Davis DS and Craig TM. 1995. Enzyme-linked immunoelectrotransfer blot analysis of excretory–secretory proteins of fascioloides magna and *Fasciola hepatica*. *Vet. Parasitol., 58: 357-363.*
- Raadsma HW, Kingsford NM, Suharyanta, Spithill TW and Piedrafita D. 2007. Host responses during experimental infection with *Fasciola gigantica* or *Fasciola hepatica* in Merino sheep I. Comparative immunological and plasma biochemical changes during early infection. *Vet. Parasitol., 143: 275-286.*
- Rabia I, Sabry H and Nagy F. 2010. Comparison between different immunological techniques for detection of circulating *Fasciola* antigen in sheep. *New York Science J., 3: 34-39.*
- Ragab FM and Farag HF. 1978. On human fascioliasis in Egypt. *J. Egy. Med. Asso., 61: 773-780.*
- Ragab FM, Mostafa BB and El-khayat HM. 2002. Influence of adjuvants on the molluscicidal activity of two plants against the intermediate hosts of schistosomiasis and fascioliasis and their toxicity to Daphnia pulex as a biological indicator. *The 2nd Cong. Rec. Techn. In Agric., Fac. Agric., Cairo Univ., Oct. 28-30, 1: 50-60.*

- **Raina OK, Sriveny D and Yadav SC. 2004.** Humotal immune response against *Fasciola gigantica* fatty acid binding protein. *Vet. Parasitol., 124: 65-72.*
- **Rajasekariah GR and Howell MJ. 1977.** The fate of *Fasciola hepatica* metacercariae following challenge infection of immune rats. *J. Helminthol., 51: 289-294.*
- **Ramajo V, Oleaga A, Casanueva P, Hillyer GV and Muro A. 2001.** Vaccination of sheep against *Fasciola hepatica* with homologous fatty acid binding proteins. *Vet. Parasitol., 97: 35-46.*
- **Reddington JJ, Leid RW and Westcott RB. 1984.** A review of antigens of *Fasciola hepatica*. *Vet. Parasitol., 14: 209-229.*
- **Richardson CD. 1994.** Expression of Thioredoxin in *Fasciola hepatica*. *Dissertation. Texas A&M University, College Station, TX.*
- **Roberts JA, Estunigsih E, Widjajanti S, Wiedosari E, Partoutomo S and Spithill TW. 1997.** Resistance of Indonesian Thin Tail sheep against Fasciola gigantica and *Fasciola hepatica*. *Vet. Parasitol., 68: 69-78.*
- **Rodriguez-Osorio M, Gomez Garcia V, Rojas J and Ramajo Martin V. 1998.** Humoral immune response and antigenemia in sheep experimentally infected with *Schistosoma bovis*. Cross-reactivity with *F. hepatica* antigens. *J. Parasitol., 85: 585-587.*
- **Rodriguez-Peréz J and Hillyer GV. 1995.** Detection of excretory-secretory circulating antigens in sheep infected with *Fasciola hepatica* and with *Schistosoma mansoni* and *Fasciola hepatica*. *Vet. Parasitol., 56: 57-66.*
- **Rothwel TLW, Windon RG, Horsburgh BA and Davies HI. 1991.** Some cutaneous responses to mitogen injection in sheep, with special reference to eosinophils leucocytes. *Res. Vet. Sci., 51: 44-47.*
- **Rottier E and Ince M. 2003.** Controlling and preventing Disease. The role of water and sanitation interventions. *Chapter: 6, pp: 74- 86.*
- **Ruis A, Molna JM, Gonzalez J, Martinez-Moreno FJ, Gutierrez PN and Martinez-Moreno A. 2003.** Humoral response (IgG) of goats experimentally infected with *Fasciola hepatica* against cysteine proteinase of adult fluke. *Vet. Res., 34: 435-443.*
- **Ruiz-Navarrete MA, Arriaga C, Bautista CR and Morilla A. 1993.** *Fasciola hepatica*: characterization of somatic and excretory-secretory antigens of adult flukes recognized by infected sheep. *Rev. Lat. Am. Microbiol., 35: 301-307.*

- **Ruth JH, Bienkowski M, Warmington KS and Lincoln PM. 1996.** IL-1 receptor antagonist (IL-1ra) expression, function, and cytokine mediated regulation during mycobacterial and schistosomal antigen-elicted granuloma formation. *J. Immunol., 156: 2503-2509.*

- **Sabry H and Mohamed S. 2007.** Diagnosis efficacy of anti-cysteine protease for detection of *Fasciola* antigen in serum and stool samples. *New Egy. J. Med., 36:163-169.*

- **Sakru N, Korkmaz M and Kuman HA. 2004.** Comparison of two different enzyme immunoassays in the diagnosis of *F. hepatica* infection. *Mikrobiyol Bul., 38: 129-135.*

- **Sampaio-Silva ML, Correia da costa JM, Viana da costa AM, Pires MA, Topes SA, Castro AM and Monjour L. 1996.** Antigenic components of excretory-secretory products of adult *F. hepatica* recognized in human infections. *Am, J. Trop. Med. Hyg., 54: 146-148.*

- **Santiago M, Hillyer GV, Garacia-Ross M and Morales MH. 1986.** Identification of functional *Fasciola hepática* antigens in experimental infections in rabbits. *Int. J. Parasitol., 14: 197-206.*

- **Savioli L, Chitsulo L and Montresor A. 1999.** New opportunities for the control of fascioliasis. *Bull. Wld. Hlth. Org., 77: 3000-3001.*

- **Schof LR, Filutowicz W, Hanna F, Juan V, Xiao BI, Mansfield N and John M. 1998.** Interleukin-4-dependant immunoglobulin G1 isotype switch in the presence of a polarized antigen-specific Th1-cell response to trypanosome variant surface glycoprotein. *Infect. Immun., 66: 451-461.*

- **Serradell MC, Guasconi L, Cervi L, Chiapello LS and Masih DT. 2007.** Excretory-secretory products from *Fasciola hepatica* induce eosinophil apoptosis by a caspase-dependent mechanism. *Vet. Immunol. Immunopathol., 117: 197-208.*

- **Sewell MMH. 1966.** The pathogenesis of fascioliasis. *Vet. Rec., 78: 98-105.*

- **Shaker ZA, Demerdash ZA, Mansour WA, Hassanein HI, EL Baz and EL Gindy HI. 1994.** Evaluation of specific Fasciola antigen in the immunodiagnosis of human fascioliasis in Egypt. *J. Egy. Soc. Parasitol., 24: 463-470.*

- **Shaker ZA, Hassanein HI, Hamed RR, Botros SS, Mahmoud FS, Mohamed SH, El-Garem AA, De Jonge N and Deelder AM. 1992.** Detection of circulating anodic antigen before and after specific chemotherapy in experimental murine *Schistosomiasis mansoni*. *Int. J. Immunopharmacol., 14: 151-158.*

- Sharma RL, Dhar DN and Raina OK. 1989. Studies on the prevalence and laboratory transmission of fascioliasis in animals in the Kashmir valley. *Brit. Vet. J., 145: 57-61.*
- Shoda LK, Rice-Ficht A, Zhu D, McKown R and Brown W. 1999. Bovine T cell responses to recombinant thioredoxin of *Fasciola hepatica*. *Vet. Parasitol., 82: 35-47.*
- Silvana C, Monica IR, Garciela S, Jorge HL, Marta GC, Enrique JB, Jorge NV, Jorge ET and Eduardo AG. 2001. Immunodiagnosis of human fascioliasis by an enzyme-linked immunosorbent assay (ELISA) and micro ELISA. *Clin. Diagn. Lab. Immunol., 8: 174-177.*
- Sinclair A and Joyner L. 1974. The effect of the aministration of a homologous antigen on the establishment of *Fasciola hepatica* in the rabbit. *Res. Vet. Sci., 16: 320-327.*
- Smith AM, Dowd AJ, McGonigle S, Keegan PS, Brennan G, Trudgett A and Dalton JP. 1993. Purification of a cathepsin L-like proteinase secreted by adult *Fasciola hepatica*. *Mol. Biochem. Parasitol., 62: 1-8.*
- Smithers SR. 1982. Fascioliasis and other trematode infections. In: Immunology of parasitic infections. Cohen S. and Warren K.S. (eds.) *Blackwell Scientific Publications, Oxford, pp. 608-621.*
- Smithers SR and Doenhoff M. 1982. Schistosomiasis. In: Immunology of Parasitic Infections. S. Cohen and S Warren. *Blackwell Scientific Publications. pp. 527-607.*
- Smyth JD. 1994. Introduction to Animal Parasitology, *third edition. Cambridge University Press, Cambridge.*
- Sobhon P, Anantavara S, Dangprasert T, Viyanant V, Krailas D, Upatham ES, Wanichanon C and Kusamran T. 1998. *Fasciola gigantica*: studies of the tegument as a basis for the developments of immunodiagnosis and vaccine. *Southeast Asian J. Trop. Med. Pub. Health., 29: 387-400.*
- Solano M, Ridley RK and Minocha HC. 1991. Production and characterization of monoclonal antibodies against excretory-secretory products of *Fasciola hepatica*. *Vet. Parasitol., 40: 227-239.*
- Soliman GN. 1996. Phylum platyhelminthes. In: Invertebrate Zoology. Soliman GN (Ed.). *The Palm Press, Zamalek, Cairo, Egypt pp. 197-201.*
- Soliman M. 2008. Epidemiological review of human and animal fascioliasis in Egypt. *J. Infect. Develop. Count., 2: 182-189.*

- **Soulsby EJL. 1973.** Helminthes: trematoda. In: Helminthes, Arthropods and Protozoa of Domesticated Animals. Soulsby EJL (Ed.). 6th edition. *Baillier, Tindall and Cssell Ltd, London, UK pp. 22-38.*
- **Soulsby EJL. 1982.** Technique. In: Helminthes, Arthropods and Protozoa of Domesticated Animals. Soulsby EJL (Ed.). 7th edition. *Bailliere Tindall, London, UK pp. 763-775.*
- **Spithill TW, Piedrafita D and Smooker PM. 1997.** Immunological approaches for the control of fascioliasis. *Int. J. Parasitol., 27: 1221-1235.*
- **Spithill TW, Smooker PM and Copeman DB. 1999a.** *Fasciola gigantica*: epidemiology, control, immunology and molecular biology. In: Fasciolosis. Dalton JP (Ed.). *CAB International publishing, Wallingford, Oxon, UK pp. 465-509.*
- **Spithill TW, Smooker PM, Sexton JI, Bozas E, Morrison CA, Creany J and Parsonf JC. 1999b.** Development of vaccine against *Fasciola hepatica*. In: fascioliasis. *Dalton, J.P. (ed) CABI Publishing Wallingford, YK. And New York, p. 377-410.*
- **Strube C, Buschbaum S, von Samson-Himmelstjerna G and Schnieder T. 2009.** Stage-dependent transcriptional changes and characterization of proteases of the bovine lungworm *Dictyocaulus viviparus*. *Parasitol. Int., 58: 334-340.*
- **Taira N, Yoshifuj H and Boray JC. 1997.** Zoonotic potential of infection with *Fasciola spp*. By consumption of freshly prepared raw liver containing immature flukes. *Int. J. Parasitol., 27: 775-779.*
- **Tantrawatpan C, Maleewong W, Wongkham C, Wongkham S, Intapan PM and Nakashima K. 2003.** Characterization of *Fasciola gigantica* adult 27-kDa excretory-secretory antigen in human fascioliasis. *Parasitol. Res., 91: 325-327.*
- **TBRI/UNEP. 1985-1987.** Research project: The effect of introducing mechanization in rice farming on transmission of schistosomiasis in Egypt. *Theodor Bilharz Research Institute, Giza, Egypt.*
- **Tijssen P and Kurstak P. 1984.** Highly efficient and simple methods for the preparation of peroxidase and active peroxidase-antibody conjugate for enzyme immunoassays. *Anal. Biochem., 136: 451-457.*
- **Timanova A, Muller S, Marti T, Bankov I and Walter RD. 1999.** Ascaridia galli fatty acid binding protein, a member of the nematode polyprotein allergens family. *Eur. J. Biochem., 261: 569-576.*

- **Tinell M, Falagiani P, Riva G and Genchi C. 1987.** RAST and ELISA in three antochonus parasitic infections in Italy: Toxariasis, Hydatidosis and fascioliasis. ***Boll.1st Sieroter, Milan., 66: 38-45.***

- **Tkalcevic J, Brandon MR and Maeusen NT. 1996.** *Fasciola hepatica*: Rapid switching of stage-specific antigen expression after infection. ***Parasitol. Immunol., 18: 139-147.***

- **Tliba O, Chauvin A, Le Vern Y, Boulard C and Sbille P. 2002.** Evaluation of the hepatic NK cell response during the early phase of *Fasciola hepatica* infection in rats. ***Vet. Res., 33: 327-332.***

- **Torgerson P and Claxton J. 1999.** Epidemiology and control. In: Fasciolosis. Dalton JP (Ed.). ***CAB International publishing, Wallingford, Oxon, UK pp 113-139.***

- **Tsang VCW, Perlata JM and Simons AR. 1983.** Enzyme-linked immunoelectrotransfer blot techniques (EITB) for studying the specificities of antigens and antibodies separated by gel electrophoresis. In: Methods in Enzymology. Immunochemical techniques. Part E.J.J. Langone and H.V. Vanakie (Eds.) New York, ***Academic Press. pp. 377-391.***

- **Ueno H and Yoshihara S. 1974.** Vertical distribution of *F. gigantica* metacercariae on stems of rice plant grown in a water pot. ***Nat. Inst. Anim. Health, 14: 54-60.***

- **Valero MA, Ubeira FM, Khoubbane M, Artigas P, Muiño L, Mezo M, Pérez-Crespo I, Periago MV and Mas-Coma S. 2009.** MM3-ELISA evaluation of coproantigen release and serum antibody production in sheep experimentally infected with *Fasciola hepatica* and *Fasciola gigantica*. ***Vet. Parasitol., 159: 77-81.***

- **Van Milligen FJ, Cornelissen JBWJ, Gaasenbeek CPH and Bokhout BA. 1998.** A novel *ex vivo* rat infection model to study protective immunity against *Fasciola hepatica* at the gut level. ***J. Immunol. Meth., 213: 183- 190.***

- **Vazquez-Talavera J, Solis CF, Medina-Escutia E, Lopez ZM, Proano J, Correa D and Laclette JP. 2001a.** Human T and B cell epitope mappining of *Taenia solium* proteases. ***Parasite Immunol., 23: 575-579.***

- **Vazquez-Talavera J, Solis CF, Terrazas LI and Laclette JP. 2001b.** Characterization and protective potential of the immune response to *Taenia solium* proteases in a murine model of cysticercosis. ***Infect. Immun., 69: 5412-5416.***

- **Velusamy R, Singh BP, Sharma RL and Chandra. 2004.** Detection of circulating 54-kDa antigen in sera of bovine calves experimentally infected with *Fasciola gigantica*. *Vet. Parasitol., 119: 187-195.*

- **Venkatesan P and Wakelin D. 1993.** ELISAs for parasitologists: or lies, damned lies and ELISAs. *Parasitol. Today, 9: 228-232.*

- **Villa-Mancera A, Quiroz-Romero H, Correa D, Ibarra F, Reyes-pe Rez M, Reyes-Vivas H, Lopez-Vela Zquez G, Gazarian K, Gazarian T and Alonso RA. 2008.** Induction of immunity in sheep to *Fasciola hepatica* with mimotopes of cathepsin L selected from a phage display library. *Parasitol., 135: 1437-1445.*

- **Voller A, Bidwell D, Huldt G and Engvall E. 1974.** A microplate method of enzyme-linked Immunosorbent assay and its application to malaria. *Bull. Wld. Health. Org., 51: 209-211.*

- **Waldvogel AS, Lepage MF, Zakher A, Reichel MP, Eicher R and Heussler VT. 2004.** Expression of interleukin 4, interleukin 4 splice variants and interferon gamma mRNA in calves experimentally infected with *Fasciola hepatica*. *Vet. Immunol. Immunopathol., 97: 53-63.*

- **Wedrychowicz H, Kesik M, Kaliniak M, Kozak-Cieszczyk M, Jedlina-Panasiuk L, Jaros S and Plucienniczak A. 2007.** Vaccine potential of inclusion bodies containing cysteine proteinase of *Fasciola hepatica* in calves and lambs experimentally challenged with metacercariae of the fluke. *Vet. Parasitol., 147: 77-88.*

- **WHO. 1995.** Control of food-borne trematode infections. WHO Exeprt Committee, Geneva, WHO Techn. Rep. No. 849.

- **WHO. 1997.** Vector control. Methods for use by individuals and communities. World Health Organization, Geneva, prepared by Dr. Jan A. Rozendal. Chapter 8: Public Health importance, food borne trematode infection (3)-freshwater snails, *p: 384-350.*

- **WHO. 2004.** Food-borne trematode infections in Asia. A Joint WHO/FAO workshop. Rep. Ser No. RS/2002/GE/40(VNT).

- **WHO. 2007.** Report of the WHO Informal Meeting on use of triclabendazole in fascioliasis control. WHO/CDS/NTD/PCT/2007.1.

- **Wijffels GL, Panaccio M, Salvatore L, Wilson L, Walker ID and Spithill TW. 1994a.** The secreted Cathepsin L-like proteinase of the trematode. *Fasciola hepatica*, contain 3-hydroxyproline residues. ***Biochem. J., 299: 781-790.***

- **Wijffels GL, Salvatore L, Dosen M, Waddington J, Wilson L, Thompson C, Campbell N, Sexton J, Wicker J, Bowen F, Friedel T and Spithill TW. 1994b.** Vaccination of sheep with purified cysteine proteinases of *Fasciola hepatica* decreases worm fecundity. *Exp. Parasitol., 78: 132-148.*
- **Wongkham C, Tantrawatpan C, Intapan PM, Maleewong W, Wongkham S and Nakashima K. 2005.** Evaluation of immunoglobulin G subclass antibodies against recombinant *Fasciola gigantica* Cathepsin L1 in an enzyme-linked immunosorbent assay for serodiagnosis of human fasciolosis. *Clin. Diagn. Lab. Immuonol., 12: 1152-1156.*
- **Yamaguchi M, Lantz CS, Oettgen HC, Katona IM, Fleming T, Miyajima I, Pierre Kinet J and Galli SJ. 1997.** IgE enhaces mouse mast cell Fc eRI expression *in vitro* and *in vivo*: evidence for a novel amplification mechanism in IgE dependant reactions. *J. Exp. Med., 185: 663-672.*
- **Yamasaki H and Aoki T. 1993.** Cloning and sequence analysis of the major cysteine protease expressed in the trematode parasite *Fasciola spp*. *Biochem. Mol. Biol. Internat., 31: 537-542.*
- **Yamasaki H, Aoki T and Oya H. 1989.** A cystein proteinase from the liver fluke *Fasciola spp*: purification, characterization, localization and application to immunodiagnosis. *Jap. J. Parasitol., 38: 373-383.*
- **Yang J, Gu Y, Yang Y, Wei J, Wang S, Cui S, Pan J, Li Q and Zhu X. 2010.** *Trichinella spiralis*: immune response and protective immunity elicited by recombinant proteases formulated with different adjuvants. *Exp. Parasitol., 124: 403-408.*
- **Yokananth S, Ghosh S, Gupta SC, Suresh MG and Saravanan D. 2005.** Characterization of specific and cross-reacting antigens of *Fasciola gigantica* by immunoblotting. *Parasitol. Res., 97: 41-48.*
- **Yokogawa M. 1982.** Newly introduced questions concerning Paragonimus westermani. *Taiwan Yi Xue Hui Za Zhi., 81: 774-780.*
- **Yousif F, El-Emam M, Abdel Kader A, Sharaf El-Din A, El-Hommossany K and Shiff C. 1999.** Schistosomiasis in newly reclaimed areas in Egypt. 2- Pattern of transmission. *J. Egypt. Soc. Parasitol., 29: 635-648.*
- **Yousif F, El-Emam M, Abdel Kader A, Sharaf El-Din A, El-Hommossany K and Shiff C. 1998b.** Schistosomiasis in newly reclaimed areas in Egypt. 1. Distribution and

population seasonal fluctuation of intermediate host snails. *J. Egypt. Soc. Parasitol., 28: 915-928.*

- **Yousif F, Ibrahim A, Abdel Kader A and El-Bardicy S. 1998a.** Invasion of the Nile Valley by a hybrid of *Biomphalaria glabrata* and *Biomphalaria alexandrina*, snail vectors of Schistosoma mansoni in Egypt. *J. Egypt. Soc. Parasitol., 28: 569-582.*

- **Youssef FG, Mansour NS and Aziz AG. 1991.** Early diagnosis of human fascioliasis by the detection of copro-antigens using counterimmunoelectrophoresis. ***Trans. R. Soc. Trop. Med. Hyg., 85: 383-384.***

- **Zhang WY, Moreau BE, Hope JC, Howard CJ, W.Y. Huang WY. 2005.** Chauvin b. Fasciola hepatica and *Fasciola gigantica*: Comparison of cellular response to experimental infection in sheep. ***Exp. Parasitol., 111: 154–159.***

- **Zhang WY, Moreau E, Yang BZ, Li ZQ, Hope JC, Howard CJ, Huang WY and Chauvin A. 2006.** Humoral and cellular immune responses to *Fasciola gigantica* experimental infection in buffaloes. ***Res Vet Sci., 80: 299-307.***

- **Zhao Q-P, Moon S-U, Na B-K, Kim S-H, Cho S-H, Lee H-W, Kong Y, Sohn W-M, Jiang M-S and Kim T-S. 2007.** *Paragonimus westermani*: Biochemical and immunological characterizations of proteases. ***Exp. Parasitol., 115: 9-18.***

- **Zheng HJ, Tao Zheng-Hou CW and Pessens WF. 1990.** Comparison of dot-ELISA with sandwich ELISA for the detection of circulating antigens in patients with Bancroftian filariasis. ***Am. J. Trop. Med. Hyg., 42: 246–254.***

- **Zhou S, Liu S, Song G, Xu Y and Sun W. 2000.** Protective immunity induced by the full-length cDNA encoding proteases of Chinese *Schistosoma japonicum*. ***Vaccine, 18: 3196-3204.***